HOPE AND DESTINY

HOPE AND DESTINY

The Patient and Parent's Guide to Sickle Cell Disease and Sickle Cell Trait

Revised Third Edition

ALLAN F. PLATT JR., P.A.-C., M.M.SC.,
JAMES ECKMAN, M.D., AND
LEWIS HSU, M.D., PH.D.

Hilton Publishing Company • Indianapolis, Indiana

Dedication

In memory of Ingrid Whittaker-Ware, Esq., who lived and shared her hopes and fulfilled her destiny.

Hilton Publishing Company
816 Fort Wayne Avenue
Indianapolis, IN 46204
317-602-8090
www.hiltonpub.com

Notice: The information in this book is true and complete to the best of the authors' and publisher's knowledge. This book is intended only as an information reference and should not replace, countermand, or conflict with the advice given to readers by their physicians. The authors and publisher disclaim all liability in connection with the specific personal use of any and all information provided in this book.

Grant E. Mabie, Managing Editor
Karla Dougherty and Lynn Bell, Editorial Assistance
David E. Haan, Layout and Design

Publisher's Cataloging-in-Publication
(Provided by Quality Books, Inc.)

Platt, Allan F.
        Hope and destiny: the patient's and parent's guide to sickle cell disease and sickle cell trait / by Allan F. Platt and Alan Sacerdote. – 2nd ed.
        p. cm.
        Includes bibliographical references and index
        ISBN: 978-0-9841447-0-9

        1. Sickle cell anemia 2. Sickle cell anemia in children.
    I. Sacerdote, Alan. II. Title

    RC641.7.S5P56 2010   616.1'527–dc22
                                                        2010043623

Printed and bound in the United States of America

AUTHORS

Allan Platt, P.A.-C., M.M.Sc., graduated with a B.S. in Health Systems Engineering from the Georgia Institute of Technology in 1977, a B.S. in Medical Science from the Emory University School of Medicine Physician Assistant program in 1979, and an M.M.Sc. in Career Physician Assistant from Emory in 2006. From 1984 until 2004 he was Program Coordinator, and Physician Assistant at the Georgia Comprehensive Sickle Cell Center at Grady Health System, the world's first dedicated 24-hour emergency center for sickle cell patients. The center is one of the largest in the world, currently providing primary and emergency care for 1,700 sickle cell patients. He is the web designer of the Sickle Cell Information Center at www. SCInfo.org. The center won AAPA Innovations in Health Care honors in 2000. In 2002, Platt received the Paragon Teacher of the Year Award from the AAPA, and, in May 2007, the SAAPA Presidents award. He is also the co-author of *Overcoming Pain* (Hilton Publishing) and author of *Evidence-Based Medicine for PDAs: A Guide for Practice* (Bartlett and Jones).

James Eckman, M.D., is a Professor of Hematology and Medical Oncology at the Winship Cancer Institute and holds appointments as Professor of Medicine and Adjunct Professor of Pediatrics in Medical Genetics at Emory University School of Medicine. He received his medical training and was appointed to the faculty of University of Minnesota Medical School before being recruited to Emory in 1978. He was committed to establishing a sickle cell program at Grady Memorial Hospital and, after intensive state lobbying for funding in 1984, became Medical Director of the world's first 24-hour comprehensive acute care sickle cell center. Under Eckman's leadership, the Georgia Comprehensive Sickle Cell Center is currently providing comprehensive health care, anticipatory guidance, and extensive psychosocial support to more than 1,300 active and 2,500 registered adult patients followed for significant sickle cell syndromes. He is an international leader in the care of sickle cell patients and has championed newborn screening for sickle cell disease nationally. This screening has saved the lives of many children with sickle cell disease who would have died from pneumococcal sepsis if timely preventive care with oral penicillin prophylaxis were not started. It was through his efforts that Georgia instituted universal mandatory sickle cell screening for newborns in October of 1998. Listed as one of America's "Top Doctors" by Castle Connolly Medical Ltd., Eckman's dedication to public health delivery of medical services, research, and the study of blood disorders has garnered him widespread recognition, honors, and memberships on numerous national committees. He was recipient of the 2000 and 2002 National Association of Public Hospitals and Health Systems Safety Net Clinician Award, was a 1998 and 2003 finalist for the Atlanta Business Chronicle Healthcare Hero, and was honored in 2006 with a special senate resolution from the Georgia General Assembly for his work in sickle cell disease.

Lewis Hsu, M.D., Ph.D., is a pediatric hematologist and clinician-scientist, with a career focus on sickle cell disease. Dr. Hsu is committed to research because of his bedside appreciation of clinical needs of patients with sickle cell disease. He has published 40 peer-reviewed papers, mentored numerous physicians and graduate students, and contributed to four sickle cell Web sites devoted to patient education. Hsu began his career path with a combined M.D.-Ph.D. at the University of Rochester School of Medicine and Dentistry. Working on his Ph.D. in Biophysics on oxygen transport in microcirculatory networks introduced him to sickle cell disease. After pediatric residency at Yale–New Haven Hospital, he focused on sickle cell disease during fellowship training in pediatric hematology-oncology at Children's Hospital of Philadelphia. In his first faculty position at Emory University, Hsu helped build the Atlanta pediatric sickle cell clinical consortium, which was a lead participant in two landmark multicenter clinical trials: bone marrow transplantation to cure sickle cell disease and transcranial Doppler ultrasound screening to prevent stroke in pediatric sickle cell disease ("the STOP study"). He collaborated on institutional trials on metabolism and neurocognitive aspects of sickle cell disease while caring for 450 children with the disease at the Georgia Comprehensive Sickle Cell Center and while teaching medical and graduate students. Hsu then worked with the highly productive National Institutes of Health (NIH) group of Drs. Mark Gladwin, Greg Kato, and Alan Schechter; this team introduced the role of nitric oxide in the pathophysiology of hemolytic anemia, such as sickle cell disease. With sickle cell mice and clinical studies, Hsu contributed to a growing body of clinical and basic research evidence stating that low availability of nitric oxide is a major feature of the complications of sickle cell disease. He also worked with sickle cell pain researcher Dr. Carlton Dampier on multicenter studies of sickle cell vaso-occlusive pain at St. Christopher's Hospital for Children in Philadelphia. Hsu recently joined Children's National Medical Center as director of one of the largest pediatric sickle cell programs in the country, where he has been building a regional collaborative approach to clinical care, research, advocacy, and education.

CONTRIBUTORS TO EARLIER EDITIONS

Dr. Benjamin Barrah. Private practice, Brooklyn, New York.

Melissa Creary. Research associate and sickle cell patient, Atlanta, Georgia.

Heidy Dodard. College Student and sickle cell patient, Atlanta, Georgia.

Berrutha Harper. President, sickle cell parent patient group.

Dr. Gregorio Hidalgo. Attending physician in hematology-oncology at Woodhull Medical and Mental Health Center, Brooklyn, New York.

Mark L'Eplattenier, P.A. Clinical coordinator and adjunct at S.U.N.Y. Health Science Center at the Brooklyn Physician Assistant Program.

Sharon Lewis. Pre-med student at Brandeis University.

Dr. Beatrice Eleje Onyeador. Resident in internal medicine at Woodhull Medical and Mental Health Center, Brooklyn, New York.

Dr. Ehi Philip Osehobo. Practices internal medicine in East Point and Fayetteville, Georgia.

Susan S. Platt, M.D. Internal medicine provider, Atlanta, Georgia.

Michelle Rodriguez. Patient, Brooklyn, New York; scholarship student at Fashion Institute of Technology in Manhattan.

Allan Sacerdote, M.D. Chief of Adult Endocrinology, Woodhull Medical and Mental Health Center, and Clinical Associate Professor of Medicine, SUNY Health Science Center, Brooklyn.

Nancy Sacerdote. B.A., Brooklyn College; M.A., Boston University.

Ingrid Whittaker-Ware, Esq. Patient representative and lawyer.

NEW CONTRIBUTOR

"Chapter 18: Gene Therapy" is written by Betty Pace, M.D., Professor of Molecular and Cell Biology at the University of Texas at Dallas, and author of *Renaissance of Sickle Cell Disease Research in the Genome Era*.

CONTRIBUTORS FROM THE GEORGIA COMPREHENSIVE SICKLE CELL CENTER AT GRADY HEALTH CENTER, ATLANTA, GEORGIA

JoAnn Beasley, R.N. Clinical Manager, Newborn Screening Coordinator, The Georgia Comprehensive Sickle Cell Center at Grady Health System

Marietta Collins, Ph.D. Pediatric Psychologist at the Georgia Comprehensive Sickle Cell Center at Grady Health System

Beatrice Gee, M.D. Assistant Professor of Pediatric Hematology/Oncology, Morehouse School of Medicine, Attending Physician at the Georgia Comprehensive Sickle Cell Center at Grady Health System

Ann E. Haight, M.D. Assistant Professor of Pediatrics, Blood and Marrow Transplant Program, Emory University School of Medicine, Aflac Cancer Center and Blood Disorders Service, Children's Healthcare of Atlanta

Melanie Jacob, M.D., M.P.H. Assistant Professor of Hematology/Oncology, Winship Cancer Institute, Emory University School of Medicine; Attending Physician at the Georgia Comprehensive Sickle Cell Center at Grady Health System

Barbara Little, M.S.N., C.N.S. Psychiatric Nurse Specialist, The Georgia Comprehensive Sickle Cell Center at Grady Health System

Patricia Myler. Multimedia Teacher and Director, The Georgia Comprehensive Sickle Cell Center at Grady Health System

Yih-Ming Yang, M.D. Professor of Pediatrics, Associate Director and Head of Education Core, Sickle Cell Program, Division of Pediatric Hematology-Oncology, Emory University School of Medicine, Aflac Cancer Center and Blood Disorders Service, Children's Healthcare of Atlanta; Co-Director of Pediatric Program at the Georgia Comprehensive Sickle Cell Program at Grady Health System

Artwork by Donna Dent, research assistant, The Georgia Comprehensive Sickle Cell Center at Grady Health System and Emory University School of Medicine

PREFACE

. . . Tionne Watkins

I'm a true believer in keeping a positive spirit and outlook on life. How you think affects how you feel. The mind is a powerful tool. If you think sick, you'll be sick. But I didn't always think this way. I spent the first seven years of my life in and out of the hospital. I was so confused, and I had no understanding as to what was going on, not to mention that my doctor at the time had diagnosed me incorrectly.

As the years went on, my mother and I started learning how to manage my pain the best way we could: hot baths, heating pads, rest, eating right, and trying to manage stress were everyday remedies. But if the pain got too bad, off we went to the hospital again. I have a great mother—so, between her care and prayers, I got through. My mother never made me feel different from other kids and never let me feel sorry for myself.

I've always been taught to think about others and to understand that there's always someone worse off than I am. I always tried to cope with being told by my doctor that I wouldn't live past 30, that I would never have children, and that I would be disabled for the rest of my life. While those words and thoughts rang in the back of my mind, that's exactly where they stayed—back somewhere.

That future the doctor told me about didn't seem like my story. In fact, I knew in my heart it wasn't going to be my life. God has the last say in my life, and that's the way I've always felt. I'm here for a reason, and I had to figure out what that reason was. I searched for answers and tried different remedies, medications, vitamins, and herbs—and still I had no success. That road wasn't fun at all; I felt like a lab rat or some experimental guinea pig. Even though some medications made me sick, put me back in the hospital, or sometimes slowed my heart rate or put me in the intensive care unit, I thought, "I can't stop, and I won't stop; something has to work." I felt like I had to take over this disease and not let it take me over.

Now, I have control over my life. At the age of 28, I met a man named Phil Oliver. He worked at the Sickle Cell Foundation. By this time, I had become the National Spokesperson for the Sickle Cell Disease Association of America. Phil pricked my finger in a Chinese herb shop and diagnosed me with Sickle-Thal, meaning one of my parents had the SC trait and the other had Beta Thalassemia. The combination of these two genes in me gave me Sickle-Thal mixed with arthritis. To be sure, I got a second opinion from Kenneth Braunstein, a wonderful hematologist I found, who then diagnosed me with the exact same thing. I'd finally found people who could help me make a change!

One thing I've learned is you have to know your body in order to explain it to your doctor so that he or she can help you. You have to pay attention to your own health. No one knows how you feel better than you. So pay attention to your body. If your doctor doesn't have good bedside manners, then find one who does. This is important, because your doctor is the person who will help keep you healthy. So you and your doctor need to be on the same page. Never be afraid to stand up for yourself. If you don't agree, say so. It's okay to ask questions. Even though we may have the same disease, it doesn't mean we will all have the same outcome. A medication that works for one may not work for the other. Everyone's genetic history is different; therefore, we may have the same situation but a different outcome. Always research medications and diagnoses for yourself. In addition to the Internet, the library is full of books to help you. Research everything you've been told and anything you've been given. Don't just take your doctor's word; find out for yourself. You'll be surprised at the things you'll learn on your own; something you learn may even save your life.

The great thing about meeting Phil is that he taught me the natural, homeopathic way of keeping up with my health. I was skeptical after trying so many other things that didn't work. I was relieved to find that the minerals and supplements I started taking on a regular basis were helping me. They weren't cures, but they helped build up my immune system (sickle cell affects your auto-immune system), which in turn helped reduce the number of sickle cell crises. Instead of me getting sick every three months, it would be three times a year. Also, when I did have a crisis, it didn't hurt as bad or last as long anymore.

So, after a lot of life-threatening situations, I am still here, living past all expectations. I continue to take natural minerals and supplements. Yes, I do go into the hospital from time to time, but not that often. I will continue to fight and search for a cure for sickle cell disease, but until then I'm still living life to the fullest. This disease doesn't have to be a death sentence, and I'm living proof of that. Can't stop, won't stop!

Grungegirl!
Shee Ent
Fax: 404-393-1125

Contents

INTRODUCTION

. . . because the life of every creature is its blood.
—Leviticus 17:14

Sickle cell disease is an inherited, lifelong problem that is located within the red blood cells of your body. A single chemical substitution in the protein hemoglobin, inside the red cell, causes that cell to take on a hard sickle shape instead of the normal soft, stretchable, doughnut shape that allows red cells to move through your blood vessels. The sickle shape causes blood flow blockages. It also causes the red blood cell to break apart *(hemolysis)*, and this causes *anemia*, or a low red blood cell count. The body pains and other complications in people with sickle cell disease are all caused by these blockages and by anemia.

In the United States, more than 80,000 people have sickle cell disease. It is one of the most common genetic diseases in this country. (It is also a serious global problem.) Each year about 1,000 babies are born in America with sickle cell disease. It is estimated that 3.5 million Americans carry the sickle cell trait—that is, they are carriers of one sickle cell gene, though they don't have the disease themselves. That is why African Americans, who are most likely to get the disease, need to be tested for sickle cell trait. Two people carrying the trait, neither of whom suffers any symptoms, may bring into the world a child with sickle cell disease who does suffer its serious effects.

Today, however, there is much good news. Now people with sickle cell disease live longer and more productive lives, thanks to early detection, preventive medications, better education about the disease, and new treatments.

Many new advances have occurred in the last 25 years to prolong life and even to cure the disease:

- People with sickle cell disease now have a life expectancy at least into their mid-40s and 50s, due especially to new methods for preventing infections, strokes, and organ damage.
- Early detection of sickle cell through newborn screening, as well as preventive treatment, education, and therapy, improves the chances of survival from infections and spleen problems from birth to age six.
- The first effective preventive medication (hydroxyurea) recently was approved by the Food and Drug Administration. This medication has reduced by half the number of pain episodes, the need for hospitalization, and the need for transfusion. Studies now show that it prolongs life.
- Bone-marrow transplants now can cure some sickle cell children who have a brother or sister to serve as a matched donor—though only the most serious cases merit the risk of going through this procedure.
- Screening children to find those at high risk of stroke allows effective preventive treatment to stop a stroke from happening.

Despite all of this good news, more needs to be done to educate patients and healthcare providers about sickle cell diseases. Even though it is one of the most common genetic diseases in the United States, research funding for it at all levels is very low because the number of patients is small and, often, the patient's economic status is low as well.

Still, much can be accomplished by motivated people working together for a common goal. The resources in this book can empower you, the reader, to become an informed, active member of the sickle cell community and to change lives for the better.

Because sickle cell disease is genetic, because it involves blood chemistry, and because it can strike many of the body's organs, it is harder to understand than diseases that strike single parts of the body.

This book explains clearly what you need to know about sickle cell disease and trait. It is based on the many questions parents, patients, and friends have asked the staff of the Georgia Comprehensive Sickle Cell Center at Grady Memorial Hospital in Atlanta, Georgia, over a period of more than 25 years.

PATIENTS' STORIES

We have included stories written by people with sickle cell disease to describe how the disease affects different age groups. From these stories and the stories posted on the Sickle Cell Information Center Web site, you will get encouragement, instruction, and hope. You may also want to tell your own story on the Web site, *www.SCInfo. org*. The people who tell these stories—parents and people with the disease who have learned to cope with it day by day—are the true heroes of this book.

HOW TO USE THIS BOOK

You may want to use the book by addressing your questions to it. With the help of the table of contents and index, you can decide which subjects you want to explore first, and get the answers from the book. You may want to journey from cover to cover. This is a preview of what is inside:

Chapter 1 is about the cells flowing in the blood stream and how they work to maintain life.

Chapter 2 explains the different types of sickle cell disease, the worldwide distribution, some preventive tips, and some sickle cell myths.

Chapter 3 is about parenting a child with sickle cell disease, and the options for parents with sickle cell trait.

Chapter 4 is a review of the issues surrounding sickle cell trait.

Chapter 5 is about interacting with the healthcare system, the professionals you may meet, and ways to ensure the best care for your disease. Common medical tests and procedures you may encounter, such as TCD and blood transfusions, are described.

Chapter 6 is all about genetics: how it determines your eye color and your looks, and how your red blood cells are made.

Chapter 7 explains the role of genetic counselors and how they help map out the combinations of genes when you have children.

Chapters 8, 9 , 10, 11, 12, and 13 offer a journey from birth to adulthood, how sickle cell disease affects the body at different stages of life, and the best prevention steps along the way.

Chapter 14 is all about pain management and ways you can treat pain.

Chapter 15 is about managing depression, a common condition in those with a lifelong medical problem.

Chapter 16 reviews the first cure offered for sickle cell disease and why it has both good and bad issues to consider.

Chapter 17 is about the only approved preventive medication for sickle cell disease and how it can help prevent pain events and complications.

Chapter 18 is all about gene therapy; now in the research stages, it may have the potential to cure more individuals with sickle cell disease.

Chapter 19 talks about the ongoing current research to find better treatments and what you can do to get involved.

Chapter 20 is the story of how you can make a difference to help those struggling with sickle cell disease.

Chapter 21 is loaded with resources, from books to Web sites, to help you learn more.

These are exciting times for sickle cell research, new treatments, and hopefully a cure for all with this disease. Keep your hope alive, and follow your destiny.

Allan Platt, James Eckman, and Lewis Hsu
January 2011

PART ONE

THE ABCs OF SICKLE CELL DISEASE

CHAPTER ONE

Understanding the Blood

More than five quarts of blood constantly move through the pipes (blood vessels) called arteries that carry blood away from the lungs, and through the veins that carry it back to the lungs. Blood carries food, oxygen, and messages to your body's organs and removes wastes, carbon dioxide, and old cell parts for recycling. Blood also helps the body heat and cool itself. It is truly the river of life.

PLASMA

Blood is made up of three types of cells and a liquid called plasma. Plasma contains the water, sugar, salt, hormones, proteins, and minerals necessary to keep cells alive. It is the fluid that carries the cells around the body to where they are needed. Plasma is filtered by the kidney, where urine is made; the liver, where protein is made and stored; and the spleen, where germs and old cells are removed from the blood.

BLOOD CELLS

There are three types of blood cells that circulate in blood vessels: red cells, white cells, and platelets.

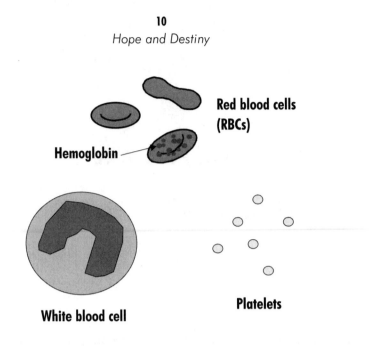

Red blood cells (RBCs)

Hemoglobin

White blood cell

Platelets

The Three Types of Blood Cells

RED CELLS

Red blood cells are the soft doughnut-shaped (the raised fluffy kind) cells. They are the "taxicabs" that carry the oxygen from your lungs to all your living cells. They pick up the waste gas, carbon dioxide, and carry it back to the lungs for you to breathe out. There are 25 trillion red blood cells in the body at any given instant. They are too small to be seen without the help of a microscope, but they give blood its red color. (For example, there would be about 50 red blood cells in the space of a period at the end of this sentence.) The red cell's shape is perfectly designed to travel the narrow capillaries out in the far parts of the body (a capillary is a tiny blood vessel that connects larger blood vessels).

Red cells normally last 120 days. Then they are destroyed in the spleen and other organs, and the chemicals that make up the cells are recycled.

The red cell is the main actor in the drama of sickle cell disease. One small change in the protein hemoglobin inside the red cell can change its shape and cause all of the problems we will talk about.

WHITE CELLS

White blood cells are the defenders of the body. They help capture and fight invading germs and protect the body against foreign cancer cells, viruses, and chemicals. There are different types of white blood cells, each with a different mission and defense location. One type of white cell makes immune protein that fights bacteria, viruses, and foreign proteins that enter the body. Other white blood cells actually eat the germs and kill bad cells. A rising white blood cell count may be the first sign of an infection attacking the body.

The white blood cells in people with sickle cell disease do not attack germs as well as they do in people without sickle cell. The result can be increased infections.

PLATELETS

Platelets are small cells that plug holes in the blood vessels. When the skin and blood vessels are cut or a hole is made, bleeding occurs. The platelets spring into action and cause the blood to form a jellylike plug, called a *clot*, to block the hole and stop the bleeding. If there are not enough platelets or they do not work right, you may not stop bleeding. If there are too many platelets, the blood may clot inside blood vessels where there is no hole. This can stop blood flow, causing damage to the tissues in the area.

Platelets are more active in people with sickle cell disease than in people without it, leading to increased clotting inside blood vessels where there is no hole.

HEMOGLOBIN

The protein inside the red blood cell that does all of the work is called *hemoglobin*. It holds the oxygen that is picked up in the lungs, releases it out into the distant tissue, and holds the carbon dioxide for a trip back to the lungs for disposal. It is the hemoglobin

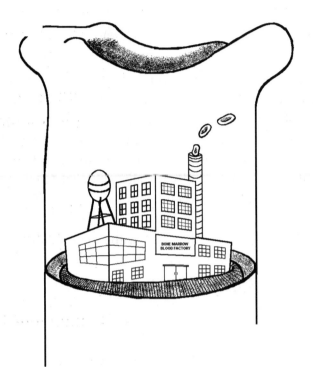

that makes the red blood cells red, and gives blood its red color. Hemoglobin with oxygen is "bright red," and hemoglobin that has given up its oxygen is "dark blue-red."

The way hemoglobin is made is determined by the DNA blueprint that every child inherits from each parent. There are normally three types of hemoglobin in each red blood cell: A, A2, and F or Fetal. Fetal hemoglobin is the main type babies have inside the womb. It tightly holds oxygen so the baby inside the womb can get the oxygen it needs from the mother's blood.

Once the baby is born, fetal hemoglobin is replaced by the adult type, hemoglobin A. Hemoglobin is made according to the genetic blueprint. Normal hemoglobin (hemoglobin A) is made up of two types of protein chains: two alpha chains and two beta chains. Trouble starts when one amino acid called *glutamic acid* on the beta chain is substituted for another called *valine*.

BONE MARROW

The red cells, white cells, and platelets are all made from stem cells in the bone marrow, inside the big bones of the body. The stem cells make the different cells needed for the blood according to the DNA, a blueprint inherited from each parent.

Anything that harms or stops the bone marrow factory can cause the red cell, white cell, and platelet number to fall, causing the person to be weak, have infections, and suffer increased bleeding.

The only cure available now for sickle cell disease is to destroy a person's bone marrow with medications and replace it, or implant it, with marrow from another person, such as a brother or sister. This changes the DNA blueprint of the blood cells to that of the donor. This is called bone marrow or stem cell transplant.

BLOOD VESSELS

Blood is carried through the miles of tubing in the body called blood vessels. The heart pumps the blood through the vessels that carry oxygenated blood from the lungs to the rest of the body. Arteries carry blood from the heart to smaller arterioles and even smaller capillaries, where the oxygen moves from the blood to the body's cells. Arteries have muscles that control blood flow and pressure by contracting to make the size of the vessel smaller or relaxing to make the opening wider. Some capillaries are smaller than the diameter of the red cell, so red cells must stretch to go through and deliver their life-giving oxygen. If the red cell becomes hard, or rigid, for any reason, it can block blood flow through the capillary.

Once the blood flows through the capillaries and delivers the oxygen, it enters tubing called the venules. The venules are another place where blood flow problems can occur in sickle cell disease. But usually blood flows from the venules and then the larger veins for its trip back to the lungs (via the heart) for more oxygen. It is in the slow-flowing venules where scientists suspect most of the sickling of the red cells occurs.

Sickled red cells are also stickier than non-sickled red cells and can become stuck to the blood vessel walls. If red cells and white cells stick abnormally to the walls of the venules, blood flow slows because cells are dammed up in the capillaries.

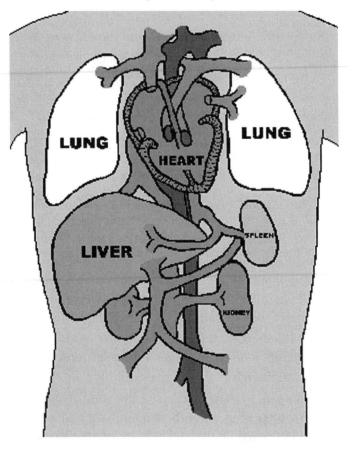

THE RED CELL CYCLE

Iron, protein, B vitamins, folate—the building blocks for red blood cells and hemoglobin—are absorbed from the food in the intestines. These nutrients are carried to the bone marrow in the middle of your large bones in the arms, legs, back, and hips. Bone marrow is the blood cell factory that makes red cells, white cells, and platelets. Infant red cells, called *reticulocytes*, are released into the blood stream and mature over two days. The red cells then are pumped around the body from the lungs to the tissues by the heart.

After its normal 120-day life, the red cell becomes easily damaged and breaks apart. The hemoglobin is released, and is broken down into a chemical called *bilirubin*. The iron and protein from the broken red cell are recycled and reused. Not eating the proper foods or any bleeding, like menstrual bleeding, can cause low iron, which can make you tired. Bleeding can also cause anemia until the body replaces the lost cells.

The kidneys also help keep red cell production going. Inside the kidneys are cells that sense the level of oxygen in the red cells. If the oxygen level is low, these cells in the kidneys secrete a hormone, called *erythropoeitin*, that travels in the blood stream to the bone marrow and stimulates more red blood cell production. It is like a call from a retail store to a factory to order more product because the shelves are empty. If the kidneys become damaged, the erythropoietin level may fall, and the bone marrow may slow down red blood cell production. This process can now be fixed with injections of manufactured erythropoietin (Epogen™, Procrit™, or Aranesp™). If doctors need to increase red blood cell production for any reason, they can boost it by giving an injection of one of these hormone replacements.

CAUSES OF ANEMIA

Anemia is a lower than normal number of red blood cells and lower hemoglobin level. Some people get anemia by not eating foods rich in iron or by not getting enough vitamins, proteins, and fats to build the red cells in the bone marrow factory. There are many causes of anemia, and it should be evaluated by your doctor.

As you know, the bone marrow factory can be attacked by infections, drugs, or chemicals, causing it to slow down production. Red blood cells can break apart before 120 days, weakening the system. This is called *hemolysis*. In sickle cell disease the red blood cells last only 15 to 20 days instead of the normal 120 days. This is the main cause of anemia in individuals with sickle cell disease. People with different types of sickle cell disease have differing severity of their anemia because of the amount of time that their red cells remain in circulation. Some people have red blood cells that break apart after five days in circulation, some after 50 days or more.

CHAPTER TWO

Sickle Cell Disease

Sickle cell is a disease caused by a change in the DNA code blueprint that alters the structure of hemoglobin. This is called a *mutation*. There are four chains in each hemoglobin molecule. Adult hemoglobin has two alpha and two beta chains. The change of one building block (called amino acids) in the beta chain alters the function of the hemoglobinmolecule, causing all the problems in the disease.

Hemoglobin is important because it delivers oxygen to all the parts of the bod. Sickle hemoglobin does not function properly because hemoglobin molecules stick together after they give up their oxygen in the small blood vessels of the body. Red cells containing sickle hemoglobin then become bent out of shape. This causes them to break apart at a young age and block the blood vessels, causing pain and other complications.

There can be many different changes in the amino acid building block structure of the hemoglobin molecule. These abnormal hemoglobins, called *hemoglobinopathies*, may cause serious disease. *Thalassemias* occur when an inherited hemoglobin problem reduces production of normal alpha or beta chains. If you carry one normal hemoglobin gene and one abnormal hemoglobin gene, you are a carrier for the disease, and may not know it because you are healthy. This is sometimes called having the "trait."

THE TYPES OF HEMOGLOBINS THAT CAUSE SICKLE CELL DISEASE

Sickle cell diseases are caused by hemoglobin (Hb) combinations, including:

- Hb SS (called sickle cell anemia);
- Hb SC;
- Hb S beta thalassemia;
- Hb SD-Punjab;
- Hb SO-Arab;
- Hb SE; and
- Hb S-HPFH (hereditary persistence of fetal hemoglobin).

Individuals with any of these combinations may have sickle complications, but some are more severe than others. Although we still don't understand why, there are many genetic differences within these hemoglobin combinations that can make one person have a milder course and some one else have a more severe disease.

HEMOGLOBIN SS—SICKLE CELL ANEMIA

Sickle cell anemia, or Hb SS, is caused by inheriting two sickle genes, one from each parent. This is the most common type of sickle cell disease.

Symptoms may include moderate to severe anemia, increased infections, tissue damage, organ damage, and recurrent pain episodes. The anemia is generally well-tolerated by patients, but the accelerated destruction of red blood cells, with increased formation of bilirubin from the released hemoglobin, does lead to a yellow color in the whites of the eyes and premature gallstones in many. Treatment with folic acid can prevent increased anemia. Blood transfusions may be needed for severe anemia and other complications. The blocked blood flow to the bones may cause pain episodes, bone infarcts (death of cell elements in the bone and marrow), and aseptic necrosis (death of tissue not caused by infection) of the hip and shoulder bones.

Sickled red blood cells can become stuck in the spleen, causing it to swell and become painful. This process of blood cells getting trapped in the spleen, along with its enlargement, is called *splenic sequestration*. Removal of the spleen for splenic sequestration is done in older children when it happens over and over.

Children and some adults may have bacterial infections that are more frequent and severe than in individuals without sickle cell disease. Tissue damage may cause pain and scarring. Strokes may occur in children because of blocked blood flow in blood vessels to the brain.Blocked blood vessels in the eye may lead to bleeding into the eye and loss of vision. As patients age, damage to the lungs causes breathing problems, and damage to the kidneys causes inability to filter toxins from the blood. Pain episodes can be unpredictable and disruptive to normal life.

HEMOGLOBIN SC

Those with Hb SC disease, the second most common type of sickle cell disease, inherit an Hb C gene from one parent and an Hb S gene from the other. In general, those with Hb SC have a sickle syndrome that is very similar to sickle cell anemia, though the hemolysis is usually less severe, so the anemia is milder. Early in life, children have fewer complications; however, adults have increased problems, making Hb SC very similar in severity to sickle cell anemia. The reported average life expectancy of those with Hb SC is in the mid-60s, compared to the mid-40s for those with Hb SS. There is a lower incidence of stroke compared to Hb SS. Having an enlarged spleen is much more common in older children and adults, though it doesn't work normally in fighting infections. This makes splenic sequestration, or the swelling of the spleen, with sickled red blood cells more common later in life than it is with sickle cell anemia. There may be more eye problems, so yearly eye examinations are required and sometimes even preventive laser surgery. Bone damage from loss of blood flow causes avascular necrosis

(AVN) of the hip and shoulder bones, and bone infarctions, making chronic pain more of a problem for older patients. Other symptoms are similar to Hb SS.

HEMOGLOBIN S BETA THALASSEMIA

Beta thalassemias are inherited disorders in the amount of hemoglobin made in red cells, caused by decreased beta globin production. In most people, the mole-cule's blueprint structure is normal, but the rate of production is reduced because of a problem communicating between the DNA blueprint to manufacturing machinery that makes the hemoglobin protein. Decreased hemoglobin production causes red blood cells to be smaller than normal and to lack hemoglobin. Beta thalassemia can combine with the sickle hemoglobin to cause sickle beta thalassemia, the third most common type of sickle cell disease.

Sickle beta thalassemia comes in two types: sickle beta^0 thalassemia and sickle beta$^+$ thalassemia. In beta^0 thalassemia there is no production of normal hemoglobin A, while in beta$^+$ thalassemia a small amount of hemoglobin A is made.

The severity of the problems related to beta thalassemia is unpredictable. Most people with sickle beta$^+$ thalassemia have working spleens and fewer problems with infection, fewer pain episodes, and less organ damage early in life. They often do very well when they get older, however, some develop complications that are as severe as in individuals with sickle cell anemia.

Those with sickle beta^0 thalassemia may have very severe disease that is almost identical to sickle cell anemia or (Hb SS). Hemoglobin levels may be higher and red blood cells smaller on average. Spleens stop working almost as early in childhood, and enlargement of the spleen is more common into than in Hb SS adulthood. Pain episodes, organ damage, and prognosis are very similar to sickle cell anemia Hb SS.

When doing genetic counseling and prenatal diagnosis for sickle cell disease, one must always consider that one partner may be a carrier of a beta thalassemia gene. These carriers are easily missed because their hemoglobin levels, common diagnostic tests, and hemoglobin electrophoresis may be normal or near normal.

HEMOGLOBIN SD, SO, SE

There are D hemoglobins that interact with Hb S, causing milder sickle cell disease with occasional pain episodes.

Hemoglobin O-Arab has significance in sickle cell disease because it interacts with Hb S to produce clinical symptoms like Hb SS disease. Hb SE sickle cell disease is not common, and cases are usually mild. The Hb E gene is very common in many areas of Southeast Asia, India, and China.

HEMOGLOBIN S-HPFH OR HEREDITARY PERSISTENCE OF FETAL HEMOGLOBIN

Hemoglobin F (fetal hemoglobin) is the main hemoglobin in the baby's red blood cells before birth. Fetal hemoglobin declines over the first six months of life. This decline is usually slower in those with sickle syndromes , and levels are slightly elevated above normal adult levels. Those with sickle cell anemia have levels from 2% to 20%, with some evidence that those with higher levels have less complications. Individuals with HPFH have high fetal hemoglobin in every red cell, and this makes the clinical problems much milder. The overall health of an individual with Hb S-HPFH is very similar to normal. The preventive medication hydroxyurea works, in part, by increasing fetal hemoglobin levels.

SICKLE HEMOGLOBIN INCIDENCE AROUND THE WORLD

In the black population in the United States, the incidence of hemoglobin S trait or sickle cell trait is approximately 8%, or about 1 in 12 individuals. The incidence of hemoglobin C trait is about 3%; and, of beta thalassemia trait, almost 1.5%. The estimates of the incidence of sickle cell syndromes are sickle cell anemia (Hb SS), 1 in every 375 live black births; sickle cell hemoglobin C disease (Hb SC), 1 in every 833 black births; and sickle cell beta thalassemia (Hb S beta-thal), 1 in every 1,667 black births.

In the Latino population in the United States, the incidence of sickle trait varies widely but averages 1 in 180 births.

THE DISTRIBUTION

Sickle cell syndromes occur in higher frequency in people from geographic areas where malaria was endemic. This occurs because carriers, like those with sickle cell trait, appear to have some protection against severe malaria infection. These genes are found most often in Africans, Arabs, Egyptians, Turks, Greeks, Italians, Iranians, and South Asians. In the United States, the disease is more common in African Americans, although it is seen in individuals of almost every ethnic background.

WORLDWIDE VIEW

Sickle cell disease is found in many countries around the world as populations have moved from place to place. Africa still has the highest incidence of trait and disease, with the incidence of sickle cell trait approaching 60% in some areas around the equator. Other territories around the world and the incidence of sickle trait are:

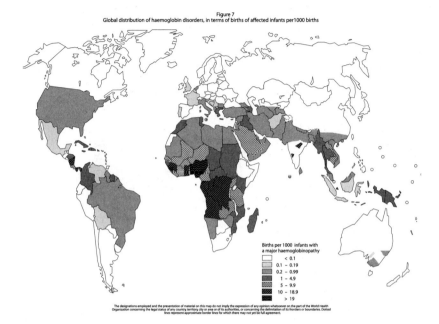

Figure 7
Global distribution of haemoglobin disorders, in terms of births of affected infants per1000 births

	Brazil 7%–10%	Puerto Rico 5%

Brazil 7%–10%
Cuba 5%
Curacao 12%
Ghana 15%
Greece 8%–27%
India 9%–38%
Jamaica 10%
Nigeria 24%

Puerto Rico 5%
Panama 12%–14%
Saudi Arabia 5%–25%
Southern Italy 10%
Surinam 15%
Venezuela 11%
West Africa 15%–25%

Incidence of Sickle Cell Disease Worldwide
http://www.who.int/genomics/public/geneticdiseases/en/index2.html#SCA

HOW SICKLE CELL DISEASE SHOWS ITSELF

People with sickle cell disease have hemoglobin that is different in only one way from that of people without sickle cell disease. This simple difference in hemoglobin is the cause of all the problems in sickle cell disease.

The difference is the way *sickle hemoglobin,* acts when it loses oxygen in the small blood vessels. Sickle hemoglobin without oxygen it forms rigid, crystal-like rods called polymers inside the red blood cells that cause cells to take on a sickle shape. Clumping of these sickled red blood cells block the blood vessels, slowing blood flow. Loss of blood flow reduces oxygen delivery (ischemia), causes body cells to die (infarction), and causes pain.

Blood cells from individuals with Hb SS are also stickier than those with Hb AA. This adds to blocking of blood flow. Platelets and white blood cells also plug up the blood vessels and fur- ther slow blood flow. All of these actions lead to sickle cell pain episodes and most other problems.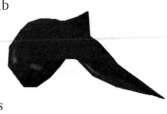

Some crises are sudden and severe; others are not. Pain episodes can be caused by low oxygen, infections, dehydration, overheating, cold exposure, your period (menses), and stress.

A newborn with sickle cell disease does not show any signs until about six months of age. The first symptom of the disorder in infants is often swelling of the hands and feet (hand-foot syndrome or *acute sickle dactylitis*). This is caused by blocked blood flow, which is caused by sickled red blood cells. This results in a rapid, painful swelling of the bone marrow cavity of the small bones in the hands and feet.

THE IMPORTANCE OF READING THE SIGNS

Nothing is more important for patients and families than to recognize the symptoms and signs of sickle cell disease complications early and start appropriate actions.

Many of the symptoms mimic those of other, more common diseases whose treatment can be quite different. For instance,

- Abdominal pain, in a sickle cell patient, might seem to be the usual pain episode related to the disease; it might, however, be due to gallstones—a condition known as *biliary colic.*
- Bone pain in a person with sickle cell disease may be mis-

taken for a typical pain episode, and the patient or family may first try pain medication at home. On the other hand, that pain could be caused by a serious bone infection known as *osteomyelitis*, which requires different treatment.

- Gallstones are more frequent in people with sickle cell disease because, as red blood cells are broken down more rapidly, they release hemoglobin, which is converted into bilirubin, which is an important component of gallstones.

In order to deal effectively with sickle cell disease you should be able to:

- recognize the typical features of a sickle cell patient;
- recognize the early signs in a previously healthy baby;
- know when to seek urgent medical attention; and
- learn to anticipate and understand the differences in appearance and development between children or siblings with sickle cell anemia and others without the disease.

Because thickening of the blood may occur anywhere in the body and cause blockages of the blood vessels, sickle cell anemia can affect a wide range of body systems. That is why complications of the disease can vary so much. Symptoms that result from any of these complications are most severe during periods called "sickle cell crisis."

PHYSICAL ISSUES

Generally, a child's final height is not affected by sickle cell disease, but the rate of growth during childhood and adolescence is slower. So final height may not be reached until the early twenties. Weight tends to be abnormally low. This may be one reason why Type 2 diabetes, which is associated strongly with obesity, is relatively rare in people with sickle cell disease, even though it is quite common in people with sickle trait. Bone development is delayed. Sexual maturation takes longer, causing delayed development

Symptoms of Sickle Cell Disease

Diagnosis	Reason for Symptoms	Symptoms
Acute Chest Syndrome	Lack of blood flow to the lungs, infection	Shortness of breath, chest pain, cough
Anemia decreased production	Increased breakdown of red blood cells, ness of breath, fainting of red blood cells	Weakness, tiredness, pale color, swelling in feet, short-
Infections	Damage to the spleen, neck pain, chest pains	Fever, severe headaches
Priapism	Lack of blood flow from the penis	Prolonged and painful erection
Stroke	Lack of blood flow to the brain or bleeding within the brain	Headache, weakness, numbness, paralysis, slurred speech, dizziness
Bone Infarction	Lack of blood supply to the bone	Severe prolonged bone pain
Splenic Sequestration	Sickled cells trapped in the spleen color	Stomach pain, swelling, weakness, tiredness, pale
Leg Ulcers	Lack of blood supply to the skin	Skin ulcers that are slow to heal
Gallstones	Make more bile stones from red blood cells breaking apart	Stomach pain, nausea, vomiting; cannot eat greasy foods
Pain Episode	Blocked blood flow to muscles and bones	Pain in the arms, legs, and back typical of past episodes
Growth and Puberty Delay	Increased calories needed	Short height, late signs of puberty
Vision— Eye Problems	Damage to blood vessels in the eye	Loss of vision, flashing lights
Swelling of Hands and Feet	Sickled cells blocking blood flow	Painful swelling of feet and hands

Unfortunately, kids and teens can be cruel, and merciless teasing about delayed growth and sexual development sometimes occurs as a result of ignorance. In severe cases of delayed growth and development, hormonal therapy with estrogen in girls or testosterone in boys may help to reverse the problem.

and onset of a period in females and delayed maturation of males' sexual organs. In severe cases of delayed growth and development, hormonal therapy may help to reverse the problem.

PSYCHOSOCIAL ISSUES

Psychosocial issues, such as depression, low self-esteem, poor family relationships, and social isolation, can arise from being chronically ill. School grades, too may be lower, if students miss many days of class. Chronic pain is a part of these childrens' lives, but, unfortunately, others sometimes misinterpret such students' reaction to pain as addictive drug-seeking behavior, or slacking off. Worse some patients *will* become addicted to pain medications. It is important to have good family support, group support, and medical care to help you with all the issues that you will face.

ECONOMIC ISSUES

The economic impact of sickle cell disease is enormous. Patients can require hospitalization for acute pain crisis, aplastic anemia, stroke, acute chest syndrome, infections, and even priapism. During hospitalization, patients will often need blood transfusions, intravenous fluid therapy, and pain management.

Careful outpatient evaluation, management, and prevention can help curb some of the cost of hospitalization. Antibiotics and immunizations can be given in the first years of life to help minimize infections. Rehabilitative services may also be required.

INFECTIONS

Infections are one of the greatest dangers to those with sickle cell disease. Bacterial infections are the most common cause of death in children during the first five years of life. Although those under three are at greatest risk for life-threatening infections, they can be acquired at any age. The spleen is the body's major defense against deadly germs. Because the spleen doesn't work properly, there is a decreased ability to fight off overwhelming infection. Serious infections such as blood infections (sepsis), infection surrounding the brain (meningitis), and lung infection (pneumonia) caused by germs are common. The bones and joints may also become infected.

Infections of the bladder and kidney are more common among people with sickle cell disease. These infections may also be more severe. Lives can be saved by detecting these infections early and treating them with the proper antibiotic. (See the section on medications within this chapter for more on this topic).

PREVENTION OF PROBLEMS: FARMS

The best way to avoid problems is to prevent them from happening. Remember FARMS—the basic principles of prevention:

F is for *Fluids and Fever*. Drink plenty of water, and manage fever. If you get a fever, see your health care provider right away.

A is for *Air*. Make sure you get enough oxygen, especially in unpressurized airplanes.

R is for *Rest*. Get plenty of sleep, do not over do it, and take plenty of breaks when your body feels tired.

M is for *prevention Medications*, like daily penicillin for children under six or hydrea for pain prevention. The vitamin Folate is needed to make new red blood cells.

S is for *Situations* to avoid, like getting too hot or cold, and avoiding smoking, alcohol, or illegal drugs.

Exercise and work outdoors wearing the proper clothing for the season. Drink plenty of water, and take frequent rest and water breaks. Carry a water bottle with you, and drink from it often. Avoid swimming pools that are too cold or hot tubs that are too hot.

Avoid emotional stress by pacing projects and work. Avoid situations that you know are upsetting. Join a support group that offers spiritual and emotional support.

FLUIDS

The simple act of consuming extra water can dramatically delay the sickling effect. Even a little bit of water can make a tremendous difference—drinking 10% more water, for example, can slow down sickling by 1,700%.

It is especially important for children with sickle cell to drink plenty of water because kidneys—along with all the other organs—are damaged by sickled cells. Once damaged, the kidneys cannot help the body retain water very well. Loss of water through urine continues at a high rate all day and all night. It is very easy for people with sickle cell to quickly become dehydrated if they do not drink enough to replace the water lost.

The best fluid is *water*. Other fluids like juice, milk, soup, fruit, or sports drinks are fine, and, to add some variety so are popsicles. On the other hand, limit drinks with *caffeine* (cola, coffee), alcohol, or theophylline, (the specific chemical which is found in tea in addition to caffeine). These ingredients make the kidney release more water into the urine. If your child is fond of cola, tea, or "energy drinks," try to limit him or her to no more than two glasses a day.

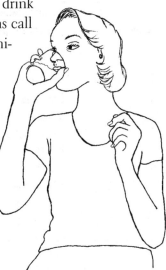

The amount of water you need to drink depends on your size. What pediatricians call the maintenance rate of fluids is the minimum you need to avoid dehydration. Half again this amount is even better.

The chart on the next page indicates how much an individual child should drink. Drinking more than the amount shown is fine, and may be necessary when the child is ill, exercising, or hot. In particular, when having sickle cell pain, make sure that he or she drinks at least the higher of the recommended amounts.

Daily Water Consumption Recommendations
Metric units version

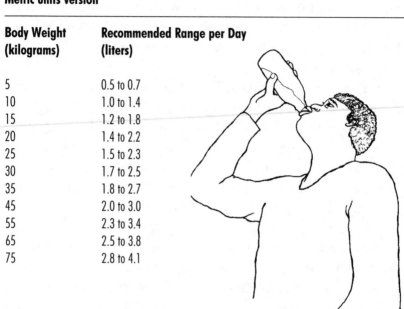

Body Weight (kilograms)	Recommended Range per Day (liters)
5	0.5 to 0.7
10	1.0 to 1.4
15	1.2 to 1.8
20	1.4 to 2.2
25	1.5 to 2.3
30	1.7 to 2.5
35	1.8 to 2.7
45	2.0 to 3.0
55	2.3 to 3.4
65	2.5 to 3.8
75	2.8 to 4.1

English units version

Body Weight (pounds)	Recommended Range per Day (8-ounce cups)
10	2 to 3 cups
25	4 to 6 cups
30	5 to 8 cups
45	6 to 9 cups
55	7 to 10 cups
75	8 to 11 cups
100	9 to 13 cups
130	10 to 15 cups
150	11 to 17 cups
175	12 to 18 cups

AIR

Air means getting enough air—and oxygen—into your lungs and into your red blood cells. The red blood cells, with sickle hemoglobin become sickled when the hemoglobin gives up its oxygen. The ways to rob the red cells of oxygen include: smoking, mountain climbing, having asthma or pneumonia, and flying in unpressurized aircraft.

You should not smoke, and, if you do, you should stop. Smoking damages lungs and robs the body of valuable oxygen. Family members who smoke should do so outside, and away from, the one with sickle cell disease. Asthma can be treated with medications that open the airways and prevent them from closing. Symptoms of shortness of breath, fever, cough, or chest pain may all be early signs of pneumonia or chest syndrome. One of the medications used to treat asthma, although not as frequently in the past, is theophylline. Because it may cause dehydration, even while improving breathing and oxygenation, its use in sickle cell patients should probably be limited to those situations where other alternatives have been exhausted, and always with good oral or intravenous hydration. If you have any of these symptons, see your doctor immediately for a complete evaluation. Do not go to higher altitudes in aircraft or hike on mountains without taking oxygen along. (See the section on air travel.)

REST

Exercising to exhaustion makes the body chemistry change to a state called *lactic acidosis*. Acidosis will often trigger sickle cell pain, and a child with a lower blood count level will reach this state sooner than one with a higher level.

To avoid exhaustion, children with sickle cell should take frequent breaks when playing. During vigorous play, taking a break every 15 to 20 minutes both to rest and to drink usually will allow them to continue their activities without developing lactic acidosis.

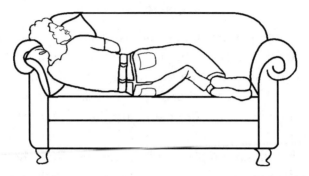

One young man, for example, often developed sickle cell pain if he played basketball for 30 minutes straight. However, he found that he could cut down on his pain episodes by playing the first quarter of a basketball game, resting the second quarter, playing the third, and resting the fourth. Physical education teachers or coaches may need a note from the family or doctor to explain this situation.

MEDICATIONS AND MEDICAL CARE

Sickle cell patients should be under the care of a medical team that understands sickle cell disease. All newborn babies with sickle cell disease should be placed on daily penicillin (or similar antibiotic) to prevent serious infections. All of the usual childhood immunizations should be given, plus the pneumococcal vaccine. Parents should know how to check for a fever, because this signals the possibility of serious infection. The following are general guidelines to keep the sickle cell patient healthy:

1. Take the vitamin folic acid (folate) daily to help make new red cells.
2. Take daily penicillin (or equivalent antibiotic) until age six to prevent serious infection.
3. Drink plenty of water daily (8–10 glasses for adults).
4. Avoid extremes of temperatures.
5. Avoid over-exertion and stress.
6. Get plenty of rest.
7. Get regular checkups from expert healthcare providers.

Patients and families should watch for the following conditions that need an urgent medical evaluation:

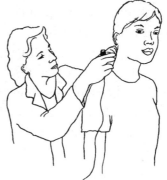

1. Fever
2. Chest pain
3. Shortness of breath
4. Increasing tiredness
5. Abdominal swelling
6. Unusual headache
7. Any sudden weakness or loss of feeling
8. Pain that will not go away with home treatment
9. Priapism (painful erection that will not go down)
10. Sudden vision change

SITUATIONS

Being either chilled or overheated changes the blood flow patterns in the body and can lead to sickle cell pain. When the weather is cold, dress your child warmly. When the weather is hot and he or she is spending time outside, make sure your child takes frequent breaks in the shade or an air-conditioned room. Many people find that swimming in unheated water can chill the body quickly and trigger sickle cell pain. That's why children with sickle cell should take rest breaks often to dry off and warm up.

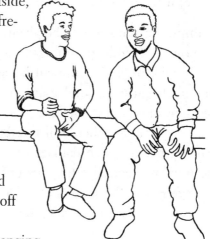

When the weather is changing quickly or your activities will take you from the hot outdoors to cool air-conditioning, make sure to dress your child in layers so that you can help regulate his or her temperature. A sweatsuit or warm-up outfit can be very helpful for staying warm before and after exercise.

Avoid using illegal drugs, such as cocaine, that are deadly to those without sickle cell disease and many times more deadly for those with it. Alcohol should also be avoided because it dehydrates the body and makes the blood more acidic—just the right conditions to increase sickling.

IMMUNIZATIONS

Because infections often trigger pain and other sickle cell crises, it is vitally important that you get immunized against certain preventable serious infections. Recommended immunizations include:

- pneumococcal (a common cause of pneumonia);
- influenza vaccine;
- hemophilus influenza type B (a common cause of sore throats, sinus and middle ear infections, acute bronchitis, and pneumonia); and
- meningococcus (a common cause of meningitis).

Immunizations should be given only when patients are in the best possible health. Immunizations should not be given when a sniffle, cold, or "flu" is present because then immunizations will more likely cause an unpleasant, or possibly dangerous, reaction. They may also be less effective.

Immunizations, should, if possible, be given when the patient is young, before much damage to the spleen has occurred. Early detection and aggressive treatment of infection is key to preventing and/or reducing the severity of sickle crises. A current listing of all recommended vaccines is available at *www.cdc.gov.*

PNEUMOCOCCAL VACCINE

Two types of pneumococcal vaccines offer protection against 90% of the strains that cause serious infection in the United States. Conjugated pneumococcal vaccine, Prevnar™, can be given as early as two months after birth, followed by two more doses six to eight weeks apart and a booster dose at 12 months. This is followed by the Pneumovax™ at ages two and five years.

MENINGOCOCCAL VACCINE

The meningococcal vaccine protects against a broad range of meningococcus strains. The meningococcal-conjugate vaccine (MCV-4) is now recommended for all children at 11–12 years of age, including those with sickle cell disease. This may be recommended for those younger than age 11 if they are exposed to someone with meningococcal infection.

Patients travelling to areas where meningococcal disease is epidemic (check with your airport's travel clinic or with the Center for Disease Control's Web site, at *www.cdc.gov*) should also receive one dose of the vaccine before leaving.

Household contacts of patients with meningococcal infection are at increased risk of infection themselves and should receive preventive treatment with the antibiotic rifampin.

For those who are unable to tolerate rifampin, there are several alternative antibiotics:

- ciprofloxaxin;
- orofloxacin; and
- ceftriaxone—for pregnant women or children under 12 years old.

Immunization for meningococcal infection is recommended not only for those who live with infected persons. It is also recommended for anyone who has had close contact with an infected patient in settings such as:

- nursery schools;
- day care centers;
- camps; . . .

. . . or for anyone who has had oral contact with an infected patient, such as kissing, mouth-to-mouth resuscitation, or sharing of the same utensil, plate, glass, cup, or toothbrush.

MALARIA PREVENTION

The prevention of malaria is complex and still controversial. What you can do for yourself is to avoid being bitten by the common Anopheles mosquito, which carries the disease.

Measures you can take:

- Avoid travel, if possible, to areas where malaria is common.
- Avoid being outdoors in such areas at peak mosquito feeding times (dusk and dawn).
- Use insect repellent regularly in such areas (increased dietary garlic and brewer's yeast have been described as excellent natural additional insect repellents).
- Wear long pants and long sleeves in endemic areas (admittedly tough in the hot tropical and subtropical areas where malaria is common).
- Use window screens.
- Use bed netting treated with the chemical permethrin (recently shown to reduce malaria deaths in Africa).

For more detailed information about malaria, see the Appendix and the CDC Web site.

LIFE EXPECTANCY

The most current information available from scientific articles is listed, and is the information we use. But keep in mind that the life expectancy keeps going up with newer treatments, better pre-

Median Survival of Individuals of All Ages with Sickle Cell Disease Based on Sickle Cell Disease Type and Sex

Sex and Genotype	Median Survival
Males with Hb SS	42 years
Females with Hb SS	48 years
Males with Hb SC	60 years
Females with Hb SC	68 years

vention, more education, genetics, healthy living, and good health care. In the Georgia Comprehensive Sickle Cell Center, we see several patients in their 50s, 60s, and 70s. We even have a 90-year-old who drops in for monitoring and treatment.

Patients should be encouraged to live every day to the fullest and prepare for a life into adulthood. Preparation should be made for work, marriage, hobbies, and meaningful contributions to society. Our patient population includes lawyers, teachers, computer programmers, artists, moms, and dads.

MYTHS EXPLODED

Myth: Sickle cell is like a cold, and you can catch it from someone with the disease.

Truth: You can not catch sickle cell disease; it is genetic. Only people who are born with this genetic defect can have it. It is lifelong and is present at birth.

Myth: You must be black to have sickle cell disease.

Truth: Sickle cell is a disease that affects people of all different racial and ethnic backgrounds, including African, Arabian, Israeli, Greek, Italian, Hispanic, Turkish, and Pakistani. The national poster child for sickle cell disease one year was a blond, blue-eyed Caucasian girl. All newborns should be screened at birth for hemoglobin traits and disease.

Myth: If our child has the disease, it means that she got the sickle cell gene from both my spouse and me.

Truth: This is true of sickle cell anemia, Hb SS, but there are other types in which only one parent has passed on the sickle cell gene and the other has passed on a gene for another type of anemia, such as Hemoglobin C, D, E, O, or thalassemia, that combine to produce sickle cell disease. This trait may be unknown to the partner.

Myth: Sickle cell trait is not important; it doesn't do anything.

Truth: Although it is a rare occurrence, sickle cell trait can cause bleeding in the urine. Under extremely severe conditions—at the limits of human endurance, such as military training or exercise at high altitude, for example—people with the trait can develop the same health problems as someone with sickle cell disease. People with sickle cell trait who also abuse alcohol may be at increased risk for a disorder of the heart muscle called alcoholic cardiomyopathy. People with trait who are also diabetic may be at an increased risk for stroke and a temporary stroke-like condition called transient ischemic attack ot TIA. Also, he or she grows up, if your child and his or her spouse both have sickle cell trait, they should be aware that their children could be born with sickle cell disease.

Myth: People with sickle cell disease or sickle cell trait cannot get malaria.

Truth: People with sickle cell disease can get malaria, and may even have a worse case. However, people with sickle cell trait tend to survive malaria better than those without the trait.

Myth: People with sickle cell will not live past the teenage years.

Truth: People with sickle cell now have a life expectancy at least into their mid-40s, thanks to several recent advances in care—in particular, new methods for preventing infections and treating fever.

Early detection of sickle cell through newborn screenings also improves survival from lung and spleen problems.

An effective medication to improve sickle cell (hydroxyurea) was approved by the Food and Drug Administration more than 10 years ago. A recent consensus conference by the National Institutes of Health concluded that hydroxyurea is used by too few people with sickle cell disease who are eligible.

Myth: There is no cure for sickle cell disease.

Truth: Nearly two hundred sickle cell patients in the United States have been cured by bone marrow transplant. The problem is this procedure needs a bone marrow donation from a genetically matched brother or sister. One must have enough complications from the disease to take the risk of the bone marrow transplant.

Myth: Sickle cell patients and their families cannot chart their own destiny.

Truth: Patients and families need to strike a balance between completely denying the presence of the disease, and living in a bubble. Learning about preventive measures and applying them can prevent complications and pain.

Myth: My child has hemoglobin SC; this is the same as sickle cell trait.

Truth: Hemoglobin SC is very definitely a type of sickle cell disease, and it has symptoms. Painful episodes for a population of children with Hb SC may not be as severe or frequent as in Hb SS (homozygous sickle cell disease), but there is wide variation between individuals. After childhood, the complications of Hb SC patients increase so that the disease becomes approximately similar in severity to adults with Hb SS. Sickle cell pain typically involves bones (including joints and skull), but can affect nearly any part of the body.

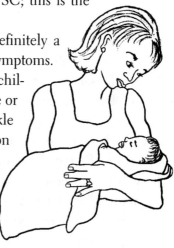

In older school-age children and adolescents with Hb SC, there is a high rate of two complications of sickle cell disease: damage to the joints (due to sickled cells interfering with blood flow to the heads of the femur and humerus), and damage to the retina of the eye (due to blocked blood vessels and abnormal growth of fragile new vessels that can bleed spontaneously). We routinely check Hb SC children for these problems, and recommend annual retinal examination by an ophthalmologist after age eight. Other sickle cell complications are less frequent in Hb SC than Hb SS (stroke, acute lung problems, aplastic crisis) but can occur.

CLIMATE

There are some reports that the mild climate of the tropics may benefit sickle cell patients. It is known that exposure to extreme cold or hot temperatures can promote sickling. Proper clothing and protection from the temperature is necessary in climates that have temperature extremes. In dry climates, drinking a lot of water is important to keep up with water losses.

SPORTS

We encourage activities that require concentration and skill rather than endurance. Golf, martial arts, skateboarding, bowling, table tennis, and fencing might be good choices. Swimming in a heated pool is also recommended because of its low impact on the hip joints. "Extreme" or endurance sports (long-distance competitive racing, for example), which push the body to exhaustion and cause dehydration, are likely to cause problems. Sports that involve cold temperatures (skiing, sky diving) or low oxygen (mountain climbing) will probably trigger sickle cell pain.

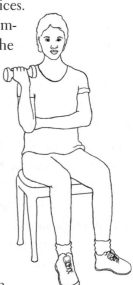

Common triggers for increased sickle cell pain are dehydration, temperature extremes (both cold and heat), low oxygen, exhaustion (lactic acidosis), infection, and stress. Sickle cell pains show up in certain places in the body because of vaso-occlusion. Generally, pain affects the long bones, the vertebrae, and the shin.

Active youngsters need to pay particular attention to the hip, where avascular necrosis is extremely common in young adults with sickle cell. This can be accelerated by repetitive injury from high-impact sports. Pain in the hip or knee should be evaluated by an orthopedist with sickle cell experience. Patients with diagnosed avascular necrosis of the hip should not participate in sports that involve repetitive jumping (basketball, dance, and gymnastics, to name a few) that may cause further injury to the hip joint.

Hydration before and during sports activity is critical. Rest breaks every 20 minutes to avoid acidosis should be scheduled.

For sprains and strains, avoid using ice. Try instead applying a cool, not cold, compress to reduce the risk of vasoconstriction, which can aggravate pain in the area.

If the patient has a very enlarged spleen, contact sports (football, hockey, lacrosse, etc.) present a risk of rupturing the organ, but the level of danger depends on the level of sports competition. Most elementary-school-age children can't hit hard enough to actually damage the spleen.

AIR TRAVEL—ALTITUDE EXPOSURE

In some patients, sickle pain episodes are caused by flying. The major problem is a decrease in oxygen in the cabin air. The aircraft is only pressurized to about 7,000 feet, which is low enough to get some people with sickle cell in trouble. The other problem is related to dehydration. The humidity in the aircraft is very low, and fluid intake needs to be markedly increased before and during the flight.

If you have had trouble flying, we would recommend supplemental oxygen at 2 liters/minute or 120 liters/hour. Most airlines are willing to provide this but require two weeks notice and a doctor's letter that establishes the need for oxygen and specifies the rate of flow.

Ask the airline for an aisle seat and plan to drink a pint of water an hour during the flight. You may wish to carry on the water you will need.

Takeoff and landing are not the critical times. The period of concern is when the plane is at greater than 10,000 feet, because that is when the cabin pressure is reduced and supplementary oxygen will be needed by the person with sickle cell.

When traveling, make sure you have a supply of all of the medicines you will need during your trip. You also should have a letter from your doctor that summarizes your disease complications and your most recent laboratory results, so that, if illness occurs, the treating doctors will know average values. Be sure all vaccinations are up to date.

Traveling to areas above 6,000 feet in elevation may cause sickle complications. Check with your doctor before going.

HEALTHY DIET, "NATURAL TREATMENTS"

While everyone needs to think about what they eat, a healthy diet is even more important for children with sickle cell disease. These key principles are good to follow:

- Children with sickle cell have the same basic nutritional requirements as anyone else.
- The food pyramid developed by the federal government is a useful guide.
- A healthy diet helps every child grow well and avoid illness.

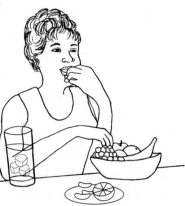

- Learning and practicing good eating habits while still young can help prevent many diseases later in life, such as heart disease, cancer, stroke, and diabetes.
- So far, researchers believe that the same antioxidants and anti-clotting foods that help prevent heart disease, stroke, and cancer also help reduce health problems caused by sickle cell disease.
- Extra fluids are very important. Avoiding dehydration is a good way to decrease the likelihood of pain crises.

Recent research shows that children with sickle cell need more calories than other children, probably 20% more at rest. Extra calories are required because of the extra energy needed to make new red blood cells. The calories contained in our fo od are converted by our bodies into energy that is used to help us grow, ward off infection, and do our daily activities. Not getting enough calories may lead to delays in growth and maturation.

Be sure your child snacks on healthy foods, such as fruits, vegetables, and grains, not just junk food. Work in some additional calories (and protein) by putting peanut butter on celery or carrots; adding cheese, nuts, or wheat germ to appropriate foods; making milkshakes or yogurt smoothies; and serving pudding or instant breakfast drinks. Many African-American and other minority youngsters and adults are lactose intolerant. They lack an intestinal enzyme called lactase, which breaks down the natural sugar in milk and dairy products called lactose. Lactose is then fermented by intestinal bacteria. Symptoms of lactose intolerance include gas pains (which may be mistaken for sickle cell–related gallbladder pain or spleen pain) and diarrhea after consuming milk or dairy products. Yogurt is the dairy product least likely to cause problems because is contains friendly bacteria called *Lactobacillus*, which have their own lactase enzyme; this removes most of the lactose from the yogurt. You can also purchase LactAid™ brand milk which has the enzyme added or take LactAid™ drops about 30 minutes before eating dairy products. The drops may also be added to normal milk to change it into LactAid™ milk, but allow at least 30 minutes for the drops to work.

Even though children with sickle cell need more calories, it is just as important for them to maintain a normal weight. Obesity can lead to faster onset of avascular necrosis of the hip, where the hip bone loses its blood supply and collapses.

Constipation may be an unfortunate side effect of some of the medications required for the treatment of sickle cell pain. Consuming plenty of fiber, such as that found in whole grains, fruits, and vegetables, will help prevent or treat constipation. When opiate pain medicines are used on a daily basis, you may need a stool softener as well as a high-fiber diet. You must drink plenty of water for these to be effective.

People with sickle cell disease need extra folic acid (also known as *folate* or *vitamin B*) to produce red blood cells more quickly. This can be found in foods such as green leafy vegetables, grains, and fresh fruits. You also should consult your child's doctor about whether or not to give a folic acid supplement and, if so, how much your child should take.

Doctors are also studying some other nutrients and foods that might aid people with sickle cell. These include omega fatty acids, magnesium, zinc, African yams, antioxidants, and certain herbs. Eating foods rich in L-Arginine like miso, yogurt, and soy protein may increase production of nitric oxide, which keeps blood vessels open. Other possible ways to increase nitric oxide may include nitrate-rich foods such as spinach and beets. Ask your doctor to keep you posted on research updates as they become available.

TEACHER/EMPLOYER GUIDE

Below is a guide that can be typed in a letter for your teachers and/ or employers. (This guide is on the Sickle Cell Information Center Web site, *www.SCInfo.org*, and can be printed directly from the site.)

- Sickle cell patients may be absent because of severe pain episodes caused by the blockage of blood flow to body organs or bones. Such episodes may require treatment in a hospital setting.
- Makeup work for students should be provided to keep the student current with assignments. A hospital or home-based teacher may be required if the student has prolonged complications.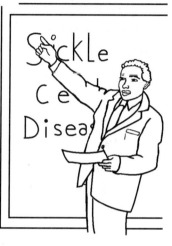
- Pain episodes may be prevented by allowing the individual to keep well hydrated with water. Do not limit the person's access to water as his or her requirements are increased. This will probably require frequent bathroom breaks.
- Pain episodes may also be prevented by not allowing the individual to become overheated or exposed to cold temperatures.
- Because of their anemia, individuals with sickle cell may tire before others, and a rest period may be appropriate. Encourage gym and sports participation, but let the person stop without undue attention.
- Sickle cell disease does not affect one's intelligence, but various factors of this lifelong illness may impair academic performance. These should be identified and addressed as they would be for any child. Because the life expectancy for those with sickle cell is now up in the fourth and fifth decade, academic performance is important. Those with sickle cell can become professionals as well as anyone else.
- Sickle cell patients may have a yellow tint to their eyes because of the anemia. They also may have a shorter stature and delayed puberty.

- Those with sickle cell should be treated as normally as possible, with an awareness that they may have intermittent episodes of pain, infection, or fatigue that can be treated and sometimes prevented, through adequate water intake, avoiding temperature extremes, and over exertion.
- Learn about sickle cell, and understand the challenges that may be faced. Have a plan of action with the individual to do what you can to keep him or her productive and complication free.

WHAT YOU CAN DO

- Invite a speaker from your local sickle cell foundation or clinic to educate the entire class or staff about sickle cell.
- Become involved in public awareness events, like walks, fun runs, kids' camp, and fund-raisers.
- Encourage blood donations and blood drives in your community. Many with sickle cell need transfusions to prevent childhood strokes and other complications.
- Support sickle cell research to provide new treatments.
- Encourage sickle cell patients to be the best they can be.

CHAPTER THREE

Raising Children Who Have Sickle Cell Disease

Train a child in the way he should go,
and when he is old he will not turn from it.
—Proverbs 22:6

Parents whose children have sickle cell disease face special problems and pressures. In this chapter, we'll talk about some of these. We'll also tell you how to work with your healthcare provider. Finally, we will make some suggestions about how to talk to your child.

WHAT IS REQUIRED OF THE PARENT

Parenting is the most rewarding job, but it is also one of the toughest. Bringing up an African-American or other minority youngster can be tougher still. While the opportunities are great for a minority child born today, the child also faces great dangers, from racism in the larger society and from the poverty, drugs, and violence that devastate many minority communities.

No wonder, then, that the parent of a child with a serious, long-term illness like sickle cell disease is often overburdened. Look at what this disease requires of such a parent:

- First, you must become a student of the disease. That means you must get to know the preventive techniques available and how to get medical help when it is needed. It also means learning to recognize and treat potential problems before they get serious.

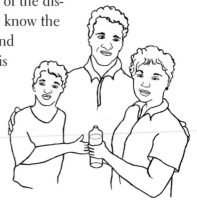

- Second, you must accept the increased financial and time commitment required to deal with the disease in your child.
- Third, you must encourage your child's growth and independence without becoming overprotective.
- Finally, if you have more than one child, you must stretch yourself to give enough attention to your healthy children. Otherwise, they are likely to become jealous of the child with sickle cell disease.

In short, sickle cell disease calls on all the parents' wisdom and love.

Sometimes, it may seem to call on more than any one human being could possibly have. Parents may feel that their own hold on ordinary life is slipping away. Careers can sink—because, just as your child is likely to experience long and frequent absences from school, you, as parent, may experience long and frequent absences from work to care for your child when he or she becomes ill.

This uncertainty may affect your choice of career, your ability to do your job well, and your chance to be promoted. Even if your company allows family leave, such policies often don't make up for lost job income.

Though family and friends often form a support community around those who suffer, parents facing their human burdens, day after day, may sometimes feel alone.

The fact is you are not alone. There are many public and private resources that can help you.

PARENTAL GUILT

Parents who pass a genetic trait that makes it more likely that he or she will have a chronic illness is likely to feel guilty. Even if you, the parents, didn't know anything about the trait before you had the child, you may be stung by the knowledge that you *could* have known. *With appropriate genetic counseling, sickle cell disease is one hundred percent preventable.* In today's climate, when it has become commonplace to ask about a lover's HIV status before becoming intimate, it should certainly be a bit easier to ask about their hemoglobin status..

Remember that it is possible for sickle cell disease to occur when only one parent has sickle trait, if the other has passed on a gene for another type of anemia, such as hemoglobin C, D, E, O, or thalassemia. This genetic combination can produce a child 25% of the time with sickle cell disease type SC, SD, SE, SO or S beta thalassemia. (See Chapter 2.)

While prevention is possible, it presents real-life problems of its own. How do you ask the person you just fell in love with to show you his or her genetic map? For that matter, how much thought do most people give to how their genes might damage a child not yet conceived? As you struggle through the problems of an everyday life, such questions may seem far away.

Even people who seek genetic counseling before they plan a family will face emotional and spiritual problems that can become crises. Especially, they must struggle to decide whether to bring a child into the world, knowing that the child may suffer from sickle cell disease. Either decision one makes can cause guilt.

ONCE YOU KNOW THE LIKELY OUTCOMES

There are strong options for parents who have had genetic counseling, who know the likely outcomes, and who still want to have a child without sickle cell disease.

ADOPTION

Some parents choose to adopt a child. Giving a home to a child who otherwise may not have one can be as fulfilling as being the biological parent. There are many agencies that can help in this process.

IN VITRO FERTILIZATION

Couples who decide to have their own biologic children can do so by using *in vitro* fertilization, also called pre-implantation genetic diagnosis (PDG). In this procedure, a sperm cell is introduced to an egg cell outside the body, in a test tube, rather than inside the body, in a Fallopian tube or in the womb. Because there is a 25% probability of a couple each with sickle cell trait having a child with sickle cell disease, the embryo is allowed to develop in the test tube until it is determined that it is free of major genetic problems, including sickle cell disease. The embryo is then implanted into the mother's womb.

In vitro fertilization is expensive, and there are limited centers that do it. But even for those who can afford it, the issues it raises can't be taken lightly. For example, the procedure requires that more than one embryo be produced in order to ensure a successful and healthy implant. While some parents can make the "test tube solution" work for them, others, because of religious or other ethical/moral concerns, cannot because it requires them to authorize the destruction of unused "test tube" embryos. Chapter seven on genetic counseling gives more details.

We've been talking as if all pregnancies were planned, but of course that isn't the case. A frequent result of an unplanned pregnancy is that you may be raising your child as a single parent. It is hard enough to raise a healthy child alone. It is far more difficult to raise a child with sickle cell disease without another loving parent to share the tears, the anxieties, the emotional and financial burdens, the time commitments, as well as the joys and triumphs. That's why it's important for all people who carry the sickle cell trait to know how to prevent sickle cell disease.

But knowledge is of little value if we don't act on it. Let's listen to one couple hashing out their problem with friends. The couple is Derrick and Laquana, and they've just been told by their genetic counselor that they carry the sickle cell trait and that they have one chance in four of having a child with sickle cell disease. The other couple, Keeshawn and Shaniqua, haven't yet been tested, but they plan to be. Laquana opens the discussion.

DERRICK AND LAQUANA'S STORY

Laquana. Derrick and I went to the doctor last week to get tested for sickle trait and other hemoglobin problems.

Derrick. Yeah, turns out we both have sickle trait.

Keeshawn. Have you decided what you'll do?

Laquana. We've thought it over a lot. Derrick wants a child, and says he's ready to be a really involved father. And you know, for me… well, we ladies do have that biological clock that keeps ticking. And I'm at the point in my career now where I can take some time off without risking my job. So we've decided to have a child.

Shaniqua. Congratulations! I'm scared about the possibility of having a child with sickle cell disease. It's hard enough to raise a normal child.

Derrick. We know it's no piece of cake. But from what the doctor told us and stuff we've been reading off the Internet, the outlook for kids with sickle cell disease is a lot better than it used to be. There are new treatments, better ways to prevent crises, even occasional cures with bone marrow transplant, and a lot more support out there for families.

Shaniqua. You know me—I have to be blunt: I just don't think it's right to bring another child into the world with a chronic illness if we can help it.

Keeshawn. Yeah, that's my feeling too. Shaniqua and I have decided that, when she gets pregnant, we'll have pre-natal testing. If the fetus tests positive for sickle cell disease, she'll have an abortion. It's not fair to bring a child into the world who's going to suffer so much, and who might have a shorter life after all that suffering.

Shaniqua. Yes. If we decide that we can't have a biological child, there are so many kids in the world who need a loving home. We can adopt one.

Laquana. Well, there you are. We feel that abortion is something we can't handle. Derrick and I will also have pre-natal testing, but if the fetus tests positive for sickle cell disease, we're going to use the rest of the pregnancy to learn as much as we can about the disease and that way give our child the longest, healthiest, happiest life possible.

Derrick. That's right. We know it won't be easy, but we've thought about it a lot. If the baby is born with sickle cell, she is going to get the best loving and caring any baby can get.

DERRICK AND LAQUANA HAVE THEIR CHILD

Derrick and Laquana went through with the plan they talked about. Throughout Laquana's pregnancy, she was carefully monitored by the pediatrician. Now the baby, Booker, is three months old and has sickle cell disease type SS. At their pediatrician's recommendation, they regularly see a pediatric hematologist at University Medical Center. They are very happy with their new pediatrician. Derrick and Laquana bring her their questions, and she takes time to explain things.

SUPPORT AND NETWORKING

As long as children with sickle cell disease do come into the world, they deserve to get the best, most loving care. By drawing on the education, support, and networking other people can provide, parents can anticipate problems and deal with them before they get too big.

One of a parent's first obligations is to know what to expect at each stage of a child's illness and so recognize problems at their earliest stages, when they can be dealt with most effectively. Managing a disease means knowing the best ways to avoid a serious outbreak of symptoms or still more serious complications. Knowing what to expect, not being caught off guard, means the parent can react earlier, in a calmer frame of mind, and prevent some emergencies.

DERRICK AND LAQUANA FIND SUPPORT

Let's tune in on Derrick and Laquana again, and see what they're up to now that their son Booker is nine months old. They are talking with their family physician.

Laquana: Booker's first crisis really shook me up. Even though we were ready for it and he got great care, he was so helpless.

Dr. Watkins: I hear what you're saying, Laquana. And I'm sorry that, the way things happened, you and Derrick had to go through it without the emotional help you might have had. Now let's correct that.

Remember a few months ago I told you that we have a sickle cell parents' support group here at the University. Over the years I've found that it really helps to talk about your experiences, fears, and solutions with other folks going through the same process. You'll meet regularly and exchange phone numbers and e-mails. Please give it some thought.

Derrick: That sounds interesting. Feeling isolated is part of the problem. I don't mean you doctors aren't helping, but sometimes we just need to talk about our feelings and our uncertainty with people who are going through what we're going through.

Dr. Watkins: I can understand that. I think you'll find what you're looking for in the parents' groups. What they do is share information. People will give you tips about something that's worked for them in dealing with a child who's hurting and scared and discouraged.

And I'm not just talking about physical pain and illness. Before long Booker will be in school. He'll want to run around with the other kids; he'll want to feel sharp in class. But there will be days

when he can't run around; days when it's
all he can do to hold his head off his
desk. Other parents can tell you how
they've been able to reassure their
own children, and what they've
said to teachers that helps.

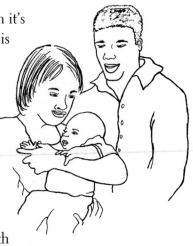

   Both of you will need comfort
and counsel yourselves. You'll
worry about medical expenses and
about time lost from work. Talking
with people who have found solutions, or at least ways of living with
tough situations—no question but that
helps.

   Sometimes you'll come away from these meetings with a new
piece of information—the name of an agency or a doctor someone
thinks highly of, or of a treatment plan that's worked. There's no end
to the resources caring people come up with when they put their
heads together to solve common problems. I'm looking forward to
hearing what you have to say about the group you join. I feel pretty
confident you'll agree it's one of the best tips I've given you.

TALKING TO YOUR CHILD

The most common problem your child may have is pain. When
your child is old enough to understand, talk to him or her about
telling you when it hurts. Love, hugs, and reassurance are great
ways to ease the pain and go a long way to quiet fears. There will be
a day when your child will want to know why he or she is different
from other children. That is the time to begin the lifelong journey
of teaching your child about sickle cell. Denying, minimizing,
ignoring, and running away from the facts will only hurt your child
in the long run. Learn all you can so you can fill your child with
life-saving knowledge. Tell your child about the blood cells. Show

pictures and drawings the child can relate to. Tell your child why it's so important to drink a lot of water, keep warm in cold weather and cool in hot weather, and how not to become over-tired. Encourage your child with play, games that challenge the mind, and reading. Limit television time, and encourage reading. Talk about careers that challenge the mind and don't strain the body.

Teaching your child openly and honestly to talk to you about pain is essential. If that communication is managed well, your child won't complain of pain in order to avoid school, homework, or chores.

Let your child know that he or she will have lots of help in being his or her best, and will have a full life ahead—as long as it is thoughtfully prepared for. There will be some stormy days, to be sure, but if the atmosphere is honest and informed, there will be far more sunny ones. Always set your expectations high for your child and teach him or her to always strive for the best even when not feeling real good.

Partner with your child's healthcare providers to learn what to discuss with your child. These specialists may offer tips, books, pictures, videos, and other materials that will make teaching fun and understandable.

Be an example for your child. What you do and how you act has a greater impact than what you say. Children follow your footsteps. If they see you calling in sick to work when you have other plans, they will repeat the pattern and use the disease as an excuse to avoid school or other responsibilities. *Be an example of responsibility, caring, giving, and hope.* This will speak volumes to your child, and you will see the seeds you have planted come to bloom in your child's life.

Take time to have family fun with outings, trips, and activities. It is critical to have the child with sickle cell disease fit into the family unit and not have the other siblings become resentful or neglected.

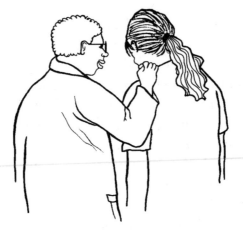

FINANCING YOUR CHILD'S CARE

Medical costs can be huge for a child with sickle cell disease. Most of the treatment programs we've talked about include social workers who will help you plan the best way to finance your child's care.

Programs like Medicaid and SCHIP are currently, available in all states and territories of the United States, as well as Puerto Rico and Washington, D.C. These can pay for practically all of your child's medical care, if you qualify. The specific requirements an individual or family must meet to qualify vary from state to state. The best source of information on your state's requirements is a social worker or the local Medicaid office.

Medicaid's stated policy now is to try to eventually force most subscribers into Medicaid-HMOs, but patients or their parents can apply for exemptions, which are usually granted, in the case of serious, chronic illnesses, like sickle cell disease.

For those who earn too much to qualify for Medicaid but who do not have insurance coverage, the options may narrow to community or county hospitals and healthcare centers. These facilities can have excellent care. Seek those hospitals affiliated with medical schools and teaching programs. This is where some of the best treatment is available. The fact is, help is available. If you don't find it at first, keep looking. You will find it eventually.

CHAPTER FOUR

Sickle Cell Trait

INCIDENCE

More than 3.5 million African Americans are carriers of sickle cell trait. This occurs , in Africa, because children with sickle trait are less likely to die when they have a malaria infection—which is a very common parasite infecting millions of people. Sickle cell trait occurs when a person inherits of just one sickle gene and one normal hemoglobin A gene. Just under half the hemoglobin inside the red blood cells is sickle hemoglobin. Young children infected with malaria parasites do not get as sick and are less likely to die because the parasite cannot grow well in the red cell with half sickle hemoglobin. Sickle hemoglobin and thalassemia are common in all parts of the world where malaria was common.

One should be certain of the diagnosis, because some people have been told they have sickle cell trait when they really have a variant of the disease. If in doubt, have the hemoglobin electrophoresis test repeated and read by a skilled hematologist. To make things more complicated, hemoglobin sickle beta$^+$ thalassemia can be misdiagnosed as sickle cell trait.

It is important to tell your healthcare providers that you have sickle cell trait. It is also important to understand some of the symptoms that can be seen under extreme conditions and how to avoid complications. Finally, knowing you have sickle cell trait means:

- You can pass this gene on to your future children.
- Sickle cell trait will never transform into sickle cell disease.
- You should have a normal life without symptoms if you avoid extremes of dehydration, very low oxygen, or extreme physical exhaustion.
- Certain occupations like flying in unpressurized aircraft, and recreational activities may cause problems.
- Travel to high altitudes can cause symptoms.

MISDIAGNOSES

If symptoms more typical of sickle cell disease, like anemia, pains, and jaundice, occur the following should be considered:

- Misdiagnosed sickle beta$^+$ thalassemia. A person with sickle beta$^+$ thalassemia may have symptoms of sickle cell disease. Always get tests and counsel from healthcare providers who understand the different types of sickle cell disease.
- Misdiagnosed sickle plus some other interacting hemoglobin like C, D, or E.
- Incorrect diagnosis. Individuals with hemoglobin SC disease are sometimes told that they have sickle trait by uninformed health professionals. This can be correctly diagnosed with a repeat hemoglobin electrophoresis.

People with sickle cell trait are generally completely normal physically and show no symptoms. Their blood evaluation is normal, with no anemia and no evidence of red cells breaking apart. There are no laboratory abnormalities other than hemoglobin AS on hemoglobin electrophoresis.

SICKLE CELL TRAIT WITH COMPLICATIONS

1. Bleeding into the urine.

a. Microscopic bleeding in the urine, or blood you cannot see in the urine without a microscope, is the most common problem experienced by people with sickle cell trait, and it only occurs in 1% to 4% of individuals with sickle trait.

b. Bloody or brown (cola colored) urine (hematuria) is very unusual. Bleeding should be evaluated by a physician, who should check for other causes. Bleeding can reoccur and can be severe enough to cause anemia. It can also cause pain if a blood clot blocks the kidney.

c. Drinking a lot of water and getting plenty of bed rest may stop pain episodes if done quickly. Bleeding may require hospital treatment with intravenous fluids and medications to slow it down.

Individuals with bleeding into the urine should drink a lot of water before, during, and after physical exertion. Those with frequent, severe, or persistent bleeding into the urine may need to avoid activities that regularly cause episodes. While blood in the urine of a patient with the sickle cell trait is probably not dangerous, the examining physician must be alert to the possibility that the bleeding comes from other, more serious causes, such as kidney or bladder stones, polyps, tumors, or bleeding disorders. A small number of people may have difficulty with recurrent blood in the urine requiring medical intervention, transfusion, and supplemental iron therapy.

VERY RARE COMPLICATIONS

1. Complications such as splenic infarction, pain episodes, and sudden death may be caused by severe cases of hypoxia and

dehydration, or by over-exertion. Fortunately, these complications are rare, and there are only sporadic case reports in the medical journals. There is no good predictor of which individuals with sickle cell trait will have these complications when placed under extreme conditions.

2. Individuals with sickle trait have a higher risk of serious complications if they exercise at the extremes of human endurance. This was recently publicized by the coaches of the National Collegiate Athletic Association after a few athletes died during rigorous football practice, some with sickle trait and some of heat-stroke without sickle trait. The intensity of exercise that causes problems in sickle cell trait also may cause problems, even death, in individuals who do not have sickle trait. The risk is higher, however, in those with sickle trait. The U.S. military found a solution to this issue decades ago, and modified the military training so that no deaths occurred among military recruits. It would be reasonable to insist that NCAA and all athletic coaches should modify training methods to avoid medical complications in athletes from over-exertion.

3. Extremely low oxygen and dehydration can cause complications like blood backing up in the spleen (splenic sequestration) and painful damage to the spleen (splenic infarction) —and pain episodes may occur, though rarely. Interestingly, Caucasians with sickle cell trait may be at higher risk for these complications. Drinking a lot of water regularly and building up exercise tolerance are important preventive measures.

Pain Episode. This is pain deep in the extremities, lower back, or chest. It should be treated like a sickle cell pain episode, with intravenous hydration, bed rest, and pain medications.

Splenic Sequestration. The symptoms of splenic sequestration are:

- abdominal pain, especially in the upper-left abdominal area; or
- weakness and abdominal swelling, especially in the upper-left abdomen.

This can happen over several minutes to hours. If you are concerned about splenic sequestration, go to an emergency room and tell the medical staff that you have sickle cell trait. Splenic sequestration may not be a complication the staff is aware of if they do not see many sickle cell patients. Treatment includes blood transfusions, and potential spleen removal.

Splenic Infarction. The symptoms are pain in the left-upper stomach that increases with breathing and may go to the left shoulder. It is treated like a pain episode.

Multi-Organ Failure and Sudden Death. There have been case reports in military and sports medical journals of sudden collapse and death in individuals with sickle cell trait as a result of extreme physical activity and little hydration. In one military study of two million recruits, a 28-fold increase in unexplained exercise-related deaths occurred in those with sickle cell trait, compared to similar age, sex, and race matched non-sickle cell trait recruits. About half of these deaths were from heat illness, and the other half had no other detectable cause except sickle cell trait.

TRAVEL PRECAUTIONS

The higher you go, the more likely you may be to develop pain or other sickle cell–related problems. People with sickle cell trait may experience trouble when they go to altitudes in excess of 10,000 feet, especially with dehydration and heavy exertion—for example, with traveling to cities with high altitudes, such as Mexico City. Car travel in mountain terrains may also cause problems.

Travel in pressurized aircraft is fine. Unpressurized aircraft may cause problems.

PREVENTION OF COMPLICATIONS

- Don't push the limit of your physical endurance.
- Always drink plenty of water, and keep a water bottle with you while exercising.
- Take rest breaks to allow the body to cool down and recover from exercise.
- Always build up slowly to a desired level of exercise.
- If traveling to a higher altitude, allow a few days to acclimate your body to the pressure and oxygen differences.
- Do not exercise immediately, but acclimate yourself to the new area. Avoid exercising in the heat of the day. It is best to walk or run in the morning or evening.

Certain sports are especially risky—for example, mountain climbing, sky diving, and skiing at high elevations. Sports and occupations that cause physical exertion in the heat, pressure changes, low oxygen, or dehydration all may cause complications.

HAVING CHILDREN

If you have sickle cell trait and you are planning to have children, have your partner tested for all the hemoglobin traits (hemoglobin S, C, D, E, O arab, beta thalassemia) that can interact with your sickle gene to give your baby sickle cell disease. This can be prevented by *in vitro* fertilization, also called pre-implantation genetic diagnosis (PDG), as discussed in chapter seven on Genetic Counseling.

The main points to remember if you have sickle cell trait are:

- You may pass this gene on to your children.
- You can be sure it will never turn into sickle cell disease.
- You can have a normal life expectancy and will almost never have medical problems from the trait.
- Certain occupations and recreational activities require some extra precautions.
- Travel to very high altitudes or severe exercise in high humidity and heat, causing dehydration, can bring on symptoms.

CHAPTER FIVE

General Medical Care

You want to be sure that you and your loved ones get the best possible medical care. You can help do this by understanding not just your disease, but also the medical and non-medical teams that can help you, and the centers and agencies you can turn to for more information and support. You also need to know how best to finance the costs of health care. Finally, you need to know something about the tests the doctors use to monitor your condition and the means by which they provide new treatment when necessary. In this chapter we introduce you to this information.

THE MEDICAL TEAM
DOCTORS

Doctors who help care for sickle cell patients perform a wide variety of roles:

Generalists: You will need a primary care physician who serves to coordinate your medical home. This may be a pediatrician, internal medicine doctor, or family physician. This doctor should be most familiar with all of your needs and problems and be the leader of the team of healthcare professionals providing your care. In some programs, the sickle cell doctor will serve in this role.

Hematologists are specially trained in blood problems, including sickle cell disease. These experts in sickle cell disease usually work in sickle cell centers in major metropolitan areas.

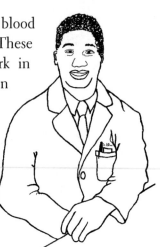

Ophthalmologists: An annual eye examination with careful evaluation of the blood vessels in the back of the eyes must be provided by a specialist familiar with sickle cell disease.

Pulmonologists treat asthma and other lung problems.

Radiologists read X-rays and scans to help diagnose problems and often place special IVs to draw blood and receive medications in the vein.

Surgeons operate on gallstones, spleens, and other conditions.

Urologists specialize in problems in the kidney and bladder needing surgery, and priapism.

Nephrologists treat kidney problems, including high blood pressure.

Obstetrician-Gynecologists care for women's health needs, administer Pap smears, and manage pregnancy.

Cardiologists treat heart problems.

Orthopedic surgeons can operate, and replace hips and shoulders damaged by avascular necrosis.

Emergency medicine specialists are staff members in emergency rooms, skilled to handle emergency situations.

Anesthesia and pain specialists provide pain management and anesthesia for surgery.

P.A.s AND N.P.s

Physician assistants (P.A.s) and nurse practitioners (N.P.s) are trained to do much of what doctors do and are supervised by doctors. P.A.s and N.P.s have special training in patient education and will spend time answering questions, doing the medical checkups, seeing patients in the hospital, and coordinating care. By handling the routine care, P.A.s and N.P.s allow the sickle cell hematologist to see more patients, especially those with more critical needs.

NURSES

Nurses provide most of the "hands on" care in the clinic, hospital, and emergency room. They are teachers, medication providers, and care coordinators. They also counsel patients and family members. Nurses are the caregivers in the hospital and are responsible for the 24-hour delivery of medications, monitoring your condition and tracking your vital signs and fluids. Nurses can be specialists in areas such as pain management or critical care, or they can be generalists. Some nurses make home visits and can administer antibiotics and pain medication in the home.

PSYCHOLOGISTS AND PSYCHIATRISTS

Psychiatrists are medical doctors with special training in the use of medications to help depression, anxiety, and emotional disorders. Psychologists, who are not physicians, provide counseling, testing, and emotional support for the same issues. Both can be very important in your care because they can help you understand your feelings about your disease and life, and teach you ways to cope with problems that occur from your disease and stresses of daily life. It is important to have access to these members of the medical team when the need arises. Sickle cell is a lifelong condition that can cause emotional stresses that require professional help.

Both psychiatrists and psychologists can teach patients how to use biofeedback, distraction, and relaxation techniques to help control pain. Psychologists can help determine the cause of school problems through testing and counseling.

SOCIAL WORKERS

Social workers are trained to help others solve issues such as insurance coverage, job and school questions, housing problems, and medical disability. Social workers are experts in local support systems and funding sources. They do crisis counseling and help families get back on their feet after setbacks. Social workers are usually employed by hospitals, sickle cell centers, and health departments. The clinic or hospital social worker should be knowledgeable about the programs available in your state.

CHAPLAINS

A healthy spiritual life is very helpful for maintaining hope and a positive outlook. Chaplains are clergy employed by hospitals and clinics to help meet the spiritual needs of patients. They are available for counseling about generalized fears, fear of death, depression, and emotional stress. Chaplains are also available to help resolve ethical questions that may arise in hospitals, clinics, and medical schools such as end-of-life issues, questions concerning clinical (human) research, and stem cell research. Many chaplains sit on hospitals' human research committees, and many have some training in psychology and social work and can help these professionals serve patients more effectively.

PAIN-MANAGEMENT SPECIALISTS/CLINICS

This diverse group of experts is an important part of the care team for patients with sickle cell disease, which is too often characterized by chronic pain with superimposed episodes of acute pain due to pain crises, splenic infarctions, and avascular bone necrosis.

This specialty is an outgrowth of anesthesia, and these experts include anesthesiologists, neurologists, sports medicine specialists, neurosurgeons, orthopedic surgeons, acupuncturists, chiropractors, acupressure therapists, biofeedback therapists, massage therapists, nutritionists, and herbalists. The best pain-management centers have staff members available from all or most of these disciplines. Unfortunately, the treatment that is selected for you may be as much a function of what your particular insurance covers as what is most medically appropriate for you.

Physical Therapists

Physical therapists are trained to help exercise and strengthen muscles and joints after surgery, injury, or bone infarction. They help train patients about *transcutaneous nerve stimulation* (TNS) to block chronic pain. They can help instruct patients about how to keep damaged hips, shoulders, and other joints from getting worse.

Vocational Rehabilitation

These members of the health-care team are experts in job training and retraining. They are aware of medical conditions like sickle cell and try to match patients with jobs that will not cause medical problems. If your job *is* causing you problems, this is the expert you want to see. In most states, having sickle cell disease qualifies you for vocational rehabilitation services, including retraining. Even better, see one of these experts before applying for a job or beginning job or career training. They are usually employed by state government or by rehabilitation programs. All states have vocational rehabilitation services. Information about each program can be found at *www.jan.wvu.edu/index.htm*.

Genetic Counselors

Genetic counselors are trained to interpret genetic lab tests and construct special family trees called *pedigrees*. They can counsel you on the risk of having a child with genetic diseases such as sickle cell and discuss all of the options that may be available to you. They are available at most university and other academic medical centers.

CLINICS

The best clinics for sickle cell patients have knowledgeable and compassionate staff members. You can get recommendations from your local hematologist. You can also find out from other sickle cell patients where they get their care and if they are happy with the care. If you do not know any patients in the area, contact the nearest sickle cell association or sickle cell center for a recommendation. An updated list of clinics, sickle cell associations, and centers by state is listed on the Sickle Cell Information Center at *www.SCInfo.org/clinics.htm*. There is also a list of large clinics in the resource section of this book.

If you have HMO insurance, you may have an assigned caregiver and clinic. The clinician may be excellent, and HMOs are usually very good at preventive care. On the other hand, your clinician may have very little sickle cell experience. Ask the clinician for a referral to a sickle cell expert near your home. If the clinician can't direct you, ask the clinic administrators to direct you to the best sickle cell care available in your community. To thrive in a managed-care environment, it is necessary to be assertive—that is, politely insistent—if you sense that your care or your child's care is not going as it should. You will often have to be proactive if you or they feel you are not getting the treatment you need.

SICKLE CELL CENTERS

Sickle cell centers offer the most comprehensive services, research programs, and diverse experience. Most of these centers are located in large cities. It may be worth your while to visit the nearest center regularly and to have a care plan developed for your local clinic and emergency room. Having such a plan in writing may go a long way toward dispelling an unfortunate stereotype held by many emergency room staff that sickle cell patients, especially young Black males, are often not truly having pain, but are merely engaging in narcotic-seeking behavior.

The doctors, nurses, social workers, psychologists, nurses, genetic counselors, hematologists and educators and other clinicians in the sickle cell centers often better understand and know the special needs of an individual with sickle cell disease. A primary care provider can meet many of your medical needs, but sickle cell patients often have special problems that make it worth the effort to see experts at one of these centers.

A list of the major sickle cell centers is in the reference section of this book and is continually updated on the Sickle Cell Information Center web site at *www.SCInfo.org*.

The sickle cell centers in Atlanta, Georgia, Hollywood, Florida, Philadelphia, Pennsylvania, Baltimore, Maryland, and many other cities have acute care facilities or day clinics to treat pain events outside of the usual emergency room. These facilities have a success rate of 80% or more in helping patients get better without having to be admitted to the hospital.

EMERGENCY ROOMS

Sickle cell patients are usually dependent on their local emergency room for pain management and emergent symptoms. But help yourself before you need the emergency room. Have your regular health care provider write up an emergency room plan with your medical history, physical findings, lab values, and medications to use for pain. Have this plan placed in a notebook in your local emergency room or in your hospital chart. Keep one copy to show the nurses and physicians in the emergency room (ER) when you do go.

You must be proactive when dealing with staff in the ER. For a particular hospital, identify *before* you need them, one or several nurse and physician champions for sickle cell patients—people who can make sure you get the proper treatment.

Free detailed sickle cell guidelines for healthcare providers are available around the clock, seven days a week, on the Sickle Cell Information Web site at *www.SCInfo.org*.

Sickle Cell Foundations

Many cities and communities have sickle cell foundations that provide sickle cell blood tests and community screening at health fairs and at high schools. These foundations can provide genetic counseling, education, scholarships, summer camps, home visits, financial aid, transportation, and support groups. Most do not provide medical services, but a few foundations have nurses and trained counselors on staff to provide limited medical care. Many of these groups know of healthcare providers in the community who have expertise and interest in sickle cell disease management.

The main national organization for the various community foundations is the Sickle Cell Disease Association of America (SCDAA). Its goal is "to find a cure and improve the quality of life for those who are afflicted and their families." The SCDAA publishes and distributes, to parents and teachers, educational materials for living and coping with sickle cell disease. The contact information is listed in the reference section of this book.

Their Web site, *www.sicklecelldisease.org*, has a listing by state of all of the member organizations and their contact information. The local office of SCDAA is a valuable resource of help and support. You may also wish to volunteer at the local office and become a resource yourself.

Cost of Care

The least expensive treatment is preventive care—regular check-ups with your sickle cell provider. This is about $300 per visit.

A sickle cell patient's biggest cost is the hospital charge for in-patient stays. The average hospital stay for a sickle cell patient is five days, at a cost of $6,500. Preventive measures that reduce the need to stay in the hospital will reduce costs dramatically.

The cost will vary city to city and hospital to hospital. Emergency visits to the local emergency room account for the next largest expense. These charges can be anywhere from $200 to $1,000 per visit. In 1,400 sickle cell patients followed at the Georgia Comprehensive Sickle Cell Center at Grady Hospital in Atlanta, Georgia, the average number of emergency visits per year is three, and the need for admission has decreased to an average of one every two years.

Medications such as penicillin and folate are inexpensive. The preventive medication, hydroxyurea, costs about $1.25 a pill, and must be taken daily. Many drug companies have patient support programs that help you get the medication if you can't afford it. These programs usually require paperwork filled out by your doctor.

Cost for lab work and x-rays can add to the bill. The most expensive test is the MRI, which runs about $1,500.

Bone marrow transplant can cost nearly $300,000. Insurance companies must approve this procedure ahead of time.

WHAT IF I DON'T HAVE INSURANCE OR MONEY TO PAY FOR CARE?

Programs like Medicaid, available to people who meet financial-eligibility requirements in all states and territories of the United States, as well as Puerto Rico and Washington, D.C., can pay for practically all of your or your child's medical care, if you qualify.

The specific requirements an individual or a family must meet to qualify for Medicaid vary from state to state. The best source of information on your state's requirements is a social worker or the local Medicaid office.

Medicaid's stated policy now is to place most subscribers into Medicaid-HMOs, but patients or their parents can apply for exemptions, which are usually granted in the case of serious, chronic illnesses like sickle cell disease.

More information about Medicaid eligibility and services can be found at *www.cms.hhs.gov/medicaid/consumer.asp.*

What If I have Insurance But Find My Options Confusing?

If your employer offers healthcare insurance, arrange to talk with someone in your personnel or benefits office who can guide you to the best available options for your child and family.

If you work for a small business and no such counseling is available, seek the advice of a social worker. Many hospitals, clinics, YMCAs/YWCAs, houses of worship, and community groups offer the services of a qualified social worker free or for a nominal charge.

If no such community-based resource exists, consider hiring an independent social worker in private practice. You can find lists of social workers with phone numbers and addresses in the Yellow Pages. Friends, neighbors, doctors, nurses, and clergy are good people to ask for referrals to social workers. Usually one or two visits with a private social worker is affordable and well worth the investment.

Knowing the Details of Your Health Plan

Whatever your health plan, it pays to read it carefully and to know its regulations. If you are denied authorization for a test or treatment that your child's doctor has ordered, *be politely assertive.* You don't have to accept a "no" from the lowest-ranking person on the authority ladder. If you're not satisfied with the answer you get, ask to speak to the next person up the ladder, and so on. *Polite persistence often carries the day.* This is especially true if you belong to a managed care plan or HMO.

Working with HMOs

HMO is the common term for health maintenance organization(s), also called managed-care plans. Such plans assign patients to a primary care provider or PCP. This provider may be a family practitioner, a pediatrician, an internist, a gynecologist, a geriatrician (a specialist in the care of older adults), a physician's assistant, or a nurse-practitioner.

The PCP is in charge of your overall care and acts as a *gate-keeper* for your medical care. That is, if you are the parent of a child with sickle cell disease, the PCP determines what tests your child will have, what treatment will be recommended, and whether a specialist should be consulted.

The guiding rule of an HMO is to keep its costs low. This means that it tends to do certain things well and other things not as well. *HMOs usually do a good job of preventive care because preventing complications saves them money.* That means they are good at making sure your child gets the proper immunizations, which is key to reducing the frequency and severity of crises. *They also, usually, do a fine job of nutritional counseling,* because good diet is important in making sure that your child grows as big and strong as the disease allows, and that the child's anemia is held in check.

But you may start to run into resistance with your HMO when it comes to treatments. Your doctor (PCP) may choose a less expensive treatment even though it might not be the most effective, have the fewest side effects, or be easiest for your child to do.

This means that the PCP may limit your child's access to a blood specialist (hematologist) because such consultations cost the HMO more money. In other cases, the PCP may prefer to put most of your child's care in the hands of a specialist rather than tie up his own limited office time in the care of a complicated case.

Some HMOs might not pay for more aggressive treatments for sickle cell disease, like bone marrow transplantation. They argue that such programs are experimental, even though their usefulness in selected patients has been well established.

If you are denied treatment or service you think you should have, remember that HMOs have an appeals process. To be sure, it is stacked in favor of the bottom line, but some victories are possible.

Working with PPOs

PPOs, or preferred provider organizations, are another kind of health plan. In this type of plan you may or may not have a PCP

as gatekeeper. Often, you can simply see any specialist who partici-
pates in the plan, *without* referral from a PCP.

Some PPOs will even pay a portion of the fees for visits to doctors
outside their network, although you will be responsible for a larger
portion of the fee than if you saw a doctor within the network.

Lately, PPOs have introduced reforms that allow tests—for
example, certain imaging procedures—that they previously did
not support. PPOs often require prior approval for procedures,
and, while their prior approval staff is usually pretty reasonable, the
extra time involved may stop some doctors from ordering tests that
require such approval.

WORKING WITH TRADITIONAL FEE-FOR-SERVICE PLANS

Traditional fee-for-service plans are the third major type of health
plan. In this type of plan, which is becoming ever rarer and more
expensive, you can see any doctor you want. After an annual
deductible (which varies from one plan to another) has been met,
the plan will pay the doctor 70% to 85% of the *approved amount* for
the doctor's services. The approved amount is usually significantly
less than the doctor's standard fees.

If your child's doctor accepts assignment, you will only be
responsible for the portion of the approved amount not paid by the
plan. If your child's doctor does not accept assignment, you will
be expected to pay the doctor directly for your child's care. The
plan will then reimburse you the usual percentage of the approved
amount.

WORKING WITH MEDICARE

Your child may be able to get Medicare coverage if he or she is
awarded social security disability. For a child to qualify, he or she
must have worked on a job that withheld social security taxes. To
qualify, your child must stop working because of his or her medi-

cal condition. Information about Medicare is available at *www.medicare.gov*.

Disability/SSI

Another social security program for the disabled is SSI. To be awarded SSI a person has to fulfill the same requirements as for social security disability, except that the applicant need never have worked. The financial award is usually less than what one receives with a disability award. This program does not lead to Medicare coverage. Sickle cell complications may not allow you to do any substantial work. You should apply online at *www.socialsecurity.gov*.

Falling through the Cracks

Some people just don't quality for any federal assistance program. A few states, however, have begun to respond to this vacuum in federal programs. New York, for instance, has a low-cost health insurance program for children called Child Health Plus, which covers many of a child's basic healthcare needs. A social worker can tell you if a similar program exists in your state.

Many sickle cell clinics will provide care to you or your child, if you are unable to pay, at reduced fees or at no charge. Many public and private voluntary hospitals will provide medical care, including high-caliber specialty care, on a sliding fee scale. Establish residence in a county with a county-supported public hospital. Check out the public health clinics in your county for preventive care and immunizations. A list of public "safety net" hospitals that provide care for low-income, uninsured patients is available at *www.naph.org*. Again, a social worker can advise you.

COMMON LAB TESTS
CBC AND RETIC COUNT

The most common blood test is the complete blood count (CBC). This is actually several blood tests combined. It lets your healthcare provider know how the cells in the blood are doing. Some tests count the number of red blood cells, white blood cells, and platelets. Others measure the *hematocrit,* which is the percentage volume of red blood cells over the total volume of blood. There is a measure called the *mean corpuscular volume* (MCV) that checks the average size of the red blood cells. If the red cells are larger than normal, it might mean you are low in folate or vitamin B_{12} or on hydroxyurea. If the red cells are smaller than normal, it may mean that you are low in iron, have a thalassemia, or have lead poisoning. The hemoglobin value is also reported.

Your healthcare provider closely monitors these blood values. Each person has his or her own normal baseline. In a person with sickle cell disease, raising or lowering the blood values can cause serious complications.

The best check to see how the bone marrow factory is doing is a test that measures brand new red blood cells, called *reticulocytes.*

The white blood cell count is important to watch because it often rises when the body is under attack by viruses or bacteria.

Platelets also may increase because of the increased bone marrow production.

BLOOD CHEMISTRY VALUES

Blood chemistry values important to know about in sickle cell disease are the LDH or *lactate dehydrogenase,* an enzyme found inside red blood cells. In sickle cell patients, this value is usually way above the normal because of the constant splitting of sickled red blood cells in 14 days (hemolysis) rather than the normal 120 days. Another chemical released from the breakup of red blood cells is indirect *bilirubin,* a by-product of hemoglobin recycling.

When bilirubin levels go above 2, the white part of the eyes becomes yellow. This is not harmful, and it comes and goes with the amount of red blood cells breaking apart.

The chemistry values ALT, AST, albumin, and alkaline phosphatase all indicate how the liver is doing. When the liver becomes irritated by infection or gallstones, these values rise.

Two other chemistry tests—the blood urea nitrogen, or BUN, and creatinine— indicate how the kidneys are doing. The higher these values, the less efficiently the kidneys are filtering toxins from the blood. Two more chemistry tests, BNP and NT-BNP, can indicate whether the heart is failing to keep up with the demands of pumping blood.

Urinalysis and Urine Protein

A urinalysis consists of multiple tests on the urine that check how the kidney is working and to see if there is blood or infection in the urinary tract. Too much protein released by the kidney into the urine is one of the first signs that the kidney has been damaged by the sickled red cells. Research is now looking for ways to prevent this damage using special blood pressure and other medications. Sickle cell patients should be screened as teenagers for protein in the urine.

Ferritin

Ferritin is the best simple blood test measure of the iron level in the body. As patients have repeated blood transfusions, iron builds up in the body. Ferratin levels indicate how much iron has built up. Iron deposits in many organs, like the liver and heart, causing damage. In order to get rid of excess iron, a medication called a chelator must be taken. In the United Sates, there are two chealtors available, Desferal® and Exjade®. A small number of sickle cell patients are low in iron, and the ferritin is an accurate test of whether there is enough iron in the body to make new red blood cells.

HEMOGLOBIN ELECTROPHORESIS

Hemoglobin electrophoresis is the blood test that determines the types of hemoglobin that are in the red blood cells. This and other methods of hemoglobin diagnosis are discussed in the diagnosis-detection chapter. Clinicians will do repeated checks of the hemoglobin S level with this test, when one is on monthly blood transfusion therapy, to make sure the treatment goals are reached.

LOOKING FOR INFECTIONS

Fever is the most important sign of infection. When clinicians suspect that an infection is present, they may order cultures of the urine, blood, throat, sputum, joint fluid, or other body fluids to see if bacteria are growing and, if so, to identify them. Cultures usually take 24–48 hours to reveal if a bacteria is present. Because waiting for the results could be deadly, an antibiotic is commonly given to protect the patient while waiting for the test results.

Other tests for infection include blood tests that detect the presence of viruses like HIV, viral hepatitis, mononucleosis, and CMV; chest and dental x-rays; bone and gallium scans; and tagged white blood cell scans. An elevated or decreased white blood cell count may be due to infection, while increased eosinophils may suggest a parasitic infestation.

COMMON PROCEDURES
IV FLUIDS

Sickle cell pain and complications can be made worse by a lack of water inside the red cells. A quick way to put the water back into the red cells is by drinking water or receiving intravenous (IV) fluids. A small plastic tube is placed in a vein, and water with 5% glucose (sugar) is allowed to drip into the blood stream. Drinking water can have the same re-hydrating effect, but it is difficult to drink enough water when pain is present.

Transfusion Therapy

Blood transfusions are necessary when the number of blood cells becomes too low, to treat or prevent a stroke, to treat acute chest syndrome, to treat splenic sequestration, and to treat persistent priapism. Transfusions are also given if the hemoglobin level is less than 10 g/dl before surgery to prevent complications. In a *simple transfusion,* a bag of donor red blood cells is dripped into a vein by an IV over a few hours. An *exchange transfusion* involves removing sickled blood cells from the person while transfusing in the donor red cells. This may be necessary in emergency situations or when the sickled red cell count is too high; the transfusion is necessary to lower the percentage of red cells containing sickle hemoglobin.

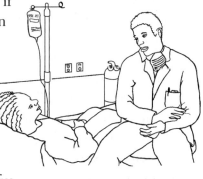

Overall, transfusions are safe. However, there are a number of important complications that may occur with transfusion. The more common important complications include too much blood volume (overload), alloimmunization, iron overload, and exposure to infections. *Fluid overload* is usually caused by doing the transfusion too quickly without the body having time to adjust to the extra red cells and fluid. This also can cause a stroke or a pain episode from the blood sludging (or becoming thick and slow flowing).

Alloimmunization is a common problem occurring in about one quarter of transfused sickle patients. The patient's immune system begins to react to the donor blood cells and attacks them. This causes a delayed transfusion reaction and development of autoantibodies, making it difficult to find a blood donor match. Prevention of alloimmunization and delayed transfusion reactions is helped by providing a record of previous transfusions, reactions, and alloantibodies to the parent and/or patient.

An alloimmunized individual should wear an identification bracelet that provides alloantibody information, a record of the best blood for the patient based on the antigens on his or her red blood cells, and a number to call to obtain the patient's transfusion history. Screening for alloantibodies six to eight weeks after transfusion will document new antibodies that may disappear if there is a prolonged period without transfusion, but still cause delayed transfusion reactions if further transfusions are required.

Limiting the number of units transfused is also important. The likelihood of causing antibodies can be reduced by using donors of the same ethnic background as the patient.

Iron overload can be prevented by limiting the amount of red blood cells transfused. Exchange transfusion, where sickled blood is removed as new donor blood is transfused in, is another method of limiting iron overload. Also, iron chelators, such as Desferal® and Exjade®, can be given to treat iron overload. Blood that is to be transfused is extensively screened for infections such as hepatitis, HIV, West Nile virus, and other infections. Individuals requiring transfusion should be immunized for hepatitis and should be tested for hepatitis (especially hepatitis C) or HIV on request. It is actually much more common to acquire these infections by way of unprotected sexual contact (especially Hepatitis B and HIV); by contaminated food or water (especially Hepatitis A or B); or by the use of street drugs by the IV, skin popping, or snorting routes, where the "works" (needles or straws) are shared or not adequately sterilized.

Testing for infectious agents markedly reduces, but does not eliminate, exposure to hepatitis, AIDS, and other viral diseases. If you received transfusions from 1975 through 1985, you should be offered counseling about the possiblility of HIV infection. Others given screened blood should be tested for hepatitis or HIV on request or in clinical situations where infection is likely.

It is extremely important for all patients and parents to carry records of all their transfusions, reactions, and alloantibodies. These should be presented to any new physician and to those giving transfusions. A running total of units transfused will help track the iron put in your body.

Whole blood thickness (viscosity), which indicates its ability to flow quickly, is often increased during complications in sickle cell disease. Transfusions are needed during certain complications because oxygen carrying is increased and the red blood cells containing sickle hemoglobin are diluted by cells with normal hemoglobin. Regular transfusions may help prevent the first or new strokes in people with sickle cell disease. Transfusions may be lifesaving during aplastic and sequestration crises.

Special considerations to be aware of when getting a transfusion are:

- exposure to infections;
- iron overload;
- too much fluid that may make blood flow slow too much; and
- developing antibodies against RBC, which makes it difficult to find matching blood.

CHELATION THERAPY FOR IRON REMOVAL

The human body holds on to iron very tightly. Iron overload occurs in people with sickle cell syndromes who have had many red cell transfusions. The body's iron stores become full after receiving approximately 20–30 transfusions. More iron accumulation beyond this point leads to problems in the heart, liver, and endocrine organs. All endocrine glands may be affected, but most commonly the pancreas (leading to diabetes mellitus) and the anterior pituitary. Pituitary problems, in turn, may cause short stature by depriving children of growth hormone; sexual, menstrual, or reproductive problems by depriving people of the gondotropins; hypoadrenalism, due to the loss of ACTH; hypothyroidism, due to the loss of TSH; and failure to produce milk for your baby after giving birth, due to the loss of prolactin.

The blood test serum ferritin is the most frequently used measure of total body iron, while hepatic iron concentration (HIC) is considered to be the most accurate measure. This test involves analyzing a sample of the liver (liver biopsy) and is done by a specialist. Magnetic resonance imaging (MRI) can estimate iron stored in heart muscle and in the liver. The superconducting quantum interference device (SQUID) can quantify iron, but there are only four machines worldwide.

Deferoxamine mesylate (Desferrioxamine, Desferal, DF) is an injectable iron remover or chelator. Iron bound to DF is excreted in the urine and turns the urine pink. DF is not well taken through the stomach and is rapidly cleared from the blood, so it is only effective for chronic chelation therapy when given through a needle for many hours a day. DF has been in regular use for treatment of transfusional iron overload since the mid-1970s. It is most frequently given using a small pump to infuse the drug under the skin over 8–12 hours at least five nights a week.

Initiation of deferoxamine therapy should be considered if, after 20–25 transfusions, *any* of the following occur:

- Transferrin saturation (Fe/TIBC ratio) is greater than 80%.
- Ferritin level is 2,000 or higher.
- Hepatic iron concentration is greater than 3 mg/gm of dry weight.

Before starting DF therapy, tests of hearing, vision, heart function, liver function, kidney function, and growth and development are recommended.

Annual reassessment of these parameters, as well as calcium metabolism and endocrine function, is suggested.

Deferoxamine (Desferal®) treatment is hard for patients to comply with, given its needles, pumps, doses, and hassle factor. The first oral iron chelator, deferiprone, was developed 20 years ago as a three-times-a-day treatment. It is less effective than deferoxamine, but it is easier to use; the side effects include joint problems and a low white blood cell count. Exjade® (ICL670, deferasirox), a once-daily oral iron chelator, was recently approved by the U.S. Food and Drug Administration. It is indicated for the treatment of chronic iron overload due to blood transfusions (transfusional hemosiderosis) in patients two years of age or older. This includes iron overload in sickle cell disease. There are other oral agents in Phase I and Phase II trials.

Exchange transfusion, or erythrocytopheresis, is a special type of blood transfusion. Blood is taken away from the body while new red blood cells are transfused. The advantages of exchange transfusion are (a) greater replacement of normal blood cells for sickle red blood cells, and (b) less iron overload. Disadvantages of exchange transfusion include: a greater exposure to red blood cell antigens, which means greater risk of alloimmunization and infection; it is more costly; and there is a greater demand on the blood bank.

ULTRASOUND

Ultrasound painlessly uses sound waves to bounce back images of body organs. It can detect gallstones, spleen size, kidney size, and if a baby is doing well in the mother's womb.

ECHOCARDIOGRAM

This particular type of ultrasound examines the heart. It can measure the size and thickness of the chambers of the heart and how well the heart muscle is squeezing. Echocardiogram can also detect backwards blood flow through one of the valves of the right heart (tricuspid valve regurgitation velocity), an important marker of possible abnormally high blood pressure in the lungs (pulmonary hypertension). The silent problem of pulmonary hypertension is important to detect by screening echocardiogram.

EXERCISE TEST AND SIX-MINUTE WALK TEST

Exercise tests can measure how well your heart and lungs are functioning. The six-minute walk test means walking back and forth in a 100-foot hallway with a hard flat surface as quickly as you can. A technician will use a stopwatch to say when six minutes are up, but is not allowed to give you coaching or encouragement. A bicycle exercise test means pedaling a stationary bike while connected to probes that measure heart rate, electrocardiogram, and oxygen level. A treadmill exercise test means walking or running on a treadmill that becomes a ramp, also while connected to probes that measure heart rate, electrocardiogram, and oxygen level. Exercise tests can be done safely with standardized techniques.

PULMONARY FUNCTION TESTS

Pulmonary function tests show how much air the lungs are moving in and out. They can indicate if a person has asthma, chronic obstructive lung disease, or reduction in lung volumes from scarring. In sickle cell disease, it's important that the lungs work well because anything that interferes with oxygen getting to the red blood cells will increase the sickling inside the body.

EYE EXAMINATIONS

Sickle cell disease, especially type SC and sickle beta$^+$ thalassemia, can cause damage to the blood vessels in the back of the eye. This can lead to bleeding and retinal detachment that causes loss of vision. The signs of early blood vessel damage can be seen by eye doctors, and treatment using lasers can prevent future damage. *We recommend that all sickle cell patients have a complete eye examination once a year to check for this early damage.*

HEARING TESTS

Sickle cell disease can cause damage to the nerves involved in hearing. Annual hearing tests are important to detect hearing loss and prevent school, work, family, and relationship problems. This is especially important if one is receiving iron chelation therapy.

TCD

Transcranial Doppler (TCD) is another painless ultrasound test that measures the speed and turbulence of blood flowing through the large blood vessels supplying the brain. When a blood vessel is about to close over because of sickle cell damage, it works a little like blocking the end of a running hose with your finger—the water comes out faster, with increased sound. The TCD is the best, nonpainful way to predict which children are at risk for having their first stroke. Such cases can be treated with blood transfusion therapy to prevent these strokes.

CT AND MRI SCANS

A computerized tomography (CT) scan is a special x-ray that allows a cross-sectional view of the organs in the body. It can detect the presence of stroke, blood, tumors, growths, swelling, and blockages within the body. Magnetic resonance imaging (MRI) uses a large, powerful magnet to make pictures of the internal organs and blood vessels. It is especially helpful in sickle cell to look for damage to the brain, certain infections, and early bone damage.

X-RAYS

The clinicians may order x-rays of the chest when looking for pneumonia or acute chest syndrome. Bone x-rays may help diagnose damage due to sickle cells or infection. This is still the most cost-effective way to look for certain complications.

BONE SCANS

Sometimes clinicians cannot tell if an infection is present in the bones. A substance that "lights-up" in areas of infection is given by IV, and the scanner traces where the substance goes. If it concentrates in one area of bone, an infection may be found that needs special treatment. Bone scans also help identify bones to repair after infarction by sickled cells blocking blood vessels to the bone.

PORTS FOR IV ACCESS

Sickle cell patients get a lot of IVs and blood tests done over the years, causing the veins to be hard and not usable. When healthcare providers must search and stick multiple places just to get blood samples and give medications and fluids, it may be time to consider a port. Ports are plastic catheters put into a large vein in the arm or chest with a small, round, quarter-sized chamber put under the skin. This chamber has a special self-sealing top that can be punctured multiple times by special bent huber needles. The port gives healthcare providers a quick and reliable access to get blood samples and give IV fluids, blood, and medications.

The good news is that, with the help of such ports, procedures usually require only one needle stick. The bad news is that these ports do not last forever because they become clotted or infected and must be replaced. This happens more commonly if they are not properly flushed or are improperly cleaned and handled. The port must be flushed with a weak heparin solution at least once a month to prevent blood from clotting within the tubing. The port must be accessed using a sterile technique to keep bacteria from getting into the port and your blood stream. It is good for you to learn all about the sterile technique and the correct needles to use to prevent healthcare providers who are not familiar with ports from causing an infection or other complications. Even with the best of care they may clot, become infected, or wear out.

IN THE HOSPITAL

If you or a family member needs to be admitted to the hospital, there are some matters that could make the stay more comfortable. If pain is a major issue, ask for a PCA (patient-controlled analgesia pump), which gives you almost complete control over the timing and dosage of pain medication. If PCA is not an option, ask your doctor to use fixed timing of the pain medication, not as needed (PRN) dosing. Addition of long-acting pain medications such as MS Contin™ or Oxycontin™ may improve pain control by maintaining a more constant amount of medication in the blood.

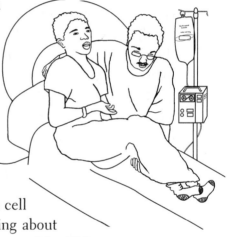

Whenever you have pain in the chest or upper stomach, or are in bed for more than a day, you should use an incentive spirometer or "blow bottle." This device exercises the lungs and prevents acute chest syndrome.

Be a teacher. Many nurses and other healthcare providers have not cared for a lot of sickle cell patients. Do some gentle teaching about the disease and its impact on your life. This will help build empathy in the workers. Some of our patients and families find that visiting the nurses on the hospital wards when they feel better and thanking them for their care goes a long way.

Keep track of fluids you drink and those you get from an IV, and track how much urine you excrete. The IV fluid of choice is D5W or sugar water. This fluid forces water into the dehydrated red blood cells and may reverse the sickling.

Get out of bed and walk as much as possible if you are able and allowed to do so.

Be sure to ask questions about what is going on, including your tests and the results.

SURGERY

If you or a family member is scheduled for surgery, here is what you need to know in order make the experience as safe as possible:

- You may need to have a simple blood transfusion to get your hemoglobin to a level of 10 g/dl. Studies have shown that this prevents postoperative complications such as acute chest syndrome. The transfusion should be given a week or two before the surgery.
- If your hemoglobin is already 10 or higher, your doctor may want to do an exchange transfusion to keep from making your blood sludge, clot, and cause complications.
- Tell the anesthesiologist (the doctor who puts you to sleep for the surgery) that you have sickle cell disease. It is important that you are kept warm, well hydrated, and well oxygenated before, during, and after the surgery to prevent a pain episode.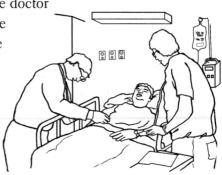
- You should be placed on an incentive spirometer or blow bottle to exercise your lungs after the surgery. This will help prevent acute chest syndrome.

INFORMATION TO KEEP

You should keep a mini-medical record of all of the important complications you have had, your medication allergies, your usual lab values, the pain medications that normally work for you, transfusion reactions and red blood cell antibodies, and your doctor's name and phone number. It is especially important to carry this information when you travel away from home, where you may have to visit a new hospital. A sample of critical information you should carry with you at all times is in the resources chapter.

CHAPTER SIX

Understanding Genetics

GENETICS AND BLOOD DISEASE

Genetics is the science that deals with heredity—that determines or reads the genetic make-up for every organ, bone, body part, and cell of your body. Your genetic make-up is like a blueprint for a building. If a builder's blueprint is wrong, it might tell the builder to put a door where a water pipe should go. If the blueprint doesn't have enough girders to hold up the building, it could collapse.

Each cell in the human body has a genetic code blueprint that tells that cell what to make and what to do. Each unit or part of the code is called a *gene*. This blueprint, or code, is passed from parents to child in the DNA in 46 chromosomes—23 from each parent. You get one half of most of your DNA code (genes or blueprint) from each of your parents. Your DNA blueprint determines your eye, hair, and skin color. It also determines your blood type and the types of the hemoglobin inside your red blood cells. A *mutation* is a change in the DNA code blueprint that can cause genetic diseases.

BLOOD TYPES

The red blood cells have antigens on the outside that are genetically determined. The main blood types are A, B, AB, and O. This blood type remains the same your entire life. There is another antigen, the Rh (Rhesus). If this is present, it will add a label of + or, if absent, a -. Your blood type may be A+, which means type "A with Rh positive, or A-, which means type A Rh negative. This is important when you need to get a blood transfusion. The blood bank will match a unit of donor blood that is compatible with your blood type. If the match is not correct, you could have a transfusion reaction, in which your body attacks the donor red cells.

There are minor red blood cell antigens such as Kell, Duffy, Diego, and Kidd. If you are exposed to several blood units over time, you may develop antibodies and have a transfusion reaction. To avoid this, the blood bank will try to match your blood to avoid the antibody-antigen reaction. Another way to prevent this is to minimize your exposure to multiple blood donors.

Laura Dean's "Blood Groups and Red Cell Antigens," a good free online book on this subject, is available at *http://www.ncbi. nlm.nih.gov/bookshelf/br.fcgi?book=rbcantigen.*

HEMOGLOBIN TYPES AND HEMOGLOBINOPATHIES

Not to be confused with ABO blood types, the hemoglobins inside the red blood cell have letters for names. The majority of the world's population has three types of hemoglobin inside each of the red cells: hemoglobin A (97%), hemoglobin F (1%), and hemoglobin A2 (2%). Your hemoglobin is genetically determined by the code on chromosomes 16 and 11. The types of hemoglobins you have can be determined by a simple blood test called the hemoglobin electrophoresis. *Hemoglobinopathies* are a group of genetic diseases that occur because of a mutation that causes a small change in the hemoglobin made in the adult red blood cell. There are more than 900 hemoglobin mutations, most without any symptoms. The substitution of the amino acid valine for glutamic acid in the sixth position of the beta chain coded on chromosome 11 causes the most famous mutation: sickle hemoglobin, or Hb S. There are other important mutations such as hemoglobin C, hemoglobin D, hemoglobin E, and hemoglobin O that can interact with sickle hemoglobin to cause sickle cell disease types SC, SD, SE, and SO. Because hemoglobin carries oxygen to all the parts of the body, the health of the hemoglobin determines the health of the body. Sickle hemoglobin is not healthy because it does not work normally after it gives up oxygen.

The structure of the hemoglobin molecule can vary widely, but variations in only one of millions of DNA coding signals can cause serious conditions, such as sickle cell disease and other diseases called *thalassemias*. Thalassemia is an inherited hemoglobin problem where not enough of the subunits (alpha or beta chains) that make up the hemoglobin structure are produced. Most hemoglobin mutations must be inherited from both parents before they cause a disease. It is possible to carry one abnormal hemoglobin gene and one normal hemoglobin gene, and not know about it because it does not show itself as disease. This is called a *carrier* state for the disease or a "trait."

SICKLE CELL TRAIT

It is generally accepted that the sickle cell mutation allowed human beings who lived in West Africa, where it first occurred, to better survive a severe infection from malaria, a red blood cell parasite. Those with sickle cell trait (one of many hemoglobin abnormalities that do not show themselves as disease) still get malaria, but they have a better chance to survive it than those without the trait. Unfortunately, the existence of the trait made the disease possible. By mating, two persons with sickle cell trait may produce offspring with sickle cell anemia (25% risk). Other hemoglobin disorders, such as beta thalassemia or hemoglobin C, may interact with sickle hemoglobin to cause a disease that is similar to sickle cell anemia. (See Chapter 4 on sickle cell trait for more details.)

It is important to tell your healthcare providers if you have sickle cell trait. It is also important for you to understand the symptoms that can show up under extreme conditions and to know how to avoid complications.

SICKLE CELL ANEMIA AND SICKLE CELL DISEASE SS

Sickle cell anemia occurs when a child inherits a gene for hemoglobin S from each parent. Both parents may have sickle trait, both may have a sickle cell disease, or one may have sickle cell trait and the other a sickle cell disease. Sickle cell anemia is a serious disease with anemia, increased infection, organ damage, and pain episodes. (See Chapter 2 for more details.)

SICKLE CELL DISEASE SC

Having the sickle cell trait can allow different combinations to form with other abnormal hemoglobins. In the one called Sickle C (SC), hemoglobin C combines with sickle cell trait. This combined version of two abnormal hemoglobins results in sickle cell disease SC, much like sickle cell disease SS, but milder in some respects.

In the situation where both parents have SC disease, there is a 25% chance of having a child with CC disease, which causes a mild anemia, occasional joint and abdominal pain, enlarged spleen, and gallstones. (See Chapter 2 for more details.)

SICKLE CELL DISEASE SE

Still another hemoglobinopathy, called hemoglobin E disease, has become common in the United States because of the large number of immigrants from Southeast Asia, where the disease originated.

In this disease, there is decreased production of hemoglobin and therefore smaller red blood cells.

This hemoglobin problem causes no anemia or other problems. Hemoglobin E can cause devastating disease when it combines with a hemoglobin problem called *thalassemia*, a most serious disease, which we discuss next. Hemoglobin E and S may combine to form sickle cell disease Hb SE. This is rare and is reported to be a milder form of sickle cell disease. (See Chapter 2 for more details.)

THALASSEMIAS AND SICKLE CELL DISEASE S BETA THALASSEMIA

The thalassemias are a group of diseases that make the body less able—or even *unable*—to use, or synthesize, one or more proteins (*globins*) that make up hemoglobin. A person who suffers from thalassemia disorder has less hemoglobin than normal available to make blood. The result can be anemia or other disorders.

Thalassemias are described as *alpha* or *beta*. Alpha thalassemia affects the alpha chain of hemoglobin, and beta thalassemia affects the beta chain of hemoglobin. While the alpha thalassemias are found primarily in people from China and Southeast Asia, they are also seen sometimes in black people. Immigration has made these diseases more common in the United States.

ALPHA THALASSEMIAS

There is a wide range of alpha thalassemias found, depending on how many of the four alpha chains in a single hemoglobin molecule get produced. When only one chain of the four is missing, the person affected is normal and won't experience (nor will the doctor detect) any signs of the disease.

At the other extreme, babies conceived with all four alpha chains (or *copies*) missing die in the womb.

Two missing alpha chains means "thalassemia minor"; the person has thalassemia trait but will live a normal life.

If there are three missing chains, a set of diseases called "hemoglobin H diseases" will develop. Hemoglobin H diseases are a serious problem because the severe breakdown of the red blood cells causes chronic anemia and an enlarged spleen.

Coexistence of sickle cell trait and alpha thalassemia trait does not result in a sickle cell disease.

BETA THALASSEMIA

Beta thalassemias result from a mutation and occur in the beta-chain manufacturing process. The mild form of beta thalassemia is called *beta thalassemia minor* because the anemia it causes is mild. Beta thalassemia minor does not require transfusion or other treatment.

People with this condition can live comfortably, but it is important that they be identified. Treating their anemia with iron, as a different kind of anemia would be treated, leads to iron overload and the deposit of iron into the body tissues.

In the severe form of beta thalassemia, termed *beta thalassemia major* or Cooley's anemia, there is little or no production of beta chains, and the hemoglobin molecule is very unstable. Individuals with this disease need frequent blood transfusions or bone marrow transplant in order to stay alive. Much of the research about iron overload and chelation therapy has come from the thalassemia patient experience.

More details about this genetic anemia can be found at *http://www.thalassemia.org*. The sickle cell community and the Cooley's anemia foundation have a lot in common and a lot to share with each other. There is strength in combining numbers when seeking funding and research support.

Beta thalassemia trait can combine with sickle cell trait to produce a type of sickle cell disease called Hb S beta thalassemia.

This can be mild to very severe, like Hb SS. (See Chapter 2 for more details.)

Beta thalassemia is common in some of the same areas as Hb S: Africa, the Mediterranean, Central and South America, India, and Pakistan. Beta thalassemia is also common in East Asia and Southeast Asia.

Another way your genetic code may affect your treatment is how you breakdown medications in your body. We know there are genetic differences in how the cytochrome P450 system in the liver works. This system works on many medications to activate them or break them down into ineffective waste products. This can cause many medications, especially the opiate class of pain medications widely used for sickle cell pain events, not to work as well. Some people will respond to small amounts of medication, while others require larger doses to get the same pain-fighting effect. There is research under way to see if we can customize the best pain treatments based on your genetic code.

Because sickle cell disease is genetic, the cure for all patients will most likely be gene therapy. More on that subject is found in Chapter 18.

CHAPTER SEVEN

Genetic Counseling

By wisdom a house is built, and through
understanding it is established.
—Proverbs 24:3

THE AIMS OF GENETIC COUNSELING

There is no cure for sickle cell anemia today except bone marrow transplants. But a couple who wishes to have children can know in advance whether their child will carry the sickle cell trait and/or actually have sickle cell disease. With that knowledge, they can prepare for the serious undertaking of raising a child with this lifelong disease. They can also consider the hard question of whether or not to bring into the world a child likely to suffer with sickle cell disease.

WHAT A GENETIC COUNSELOR DOES

A genetic counselor first:

- learns the medical history of both parents;
- orders blood tests to identify hemoglobin traits (hemoglobin-opathies) and thalassemias; and

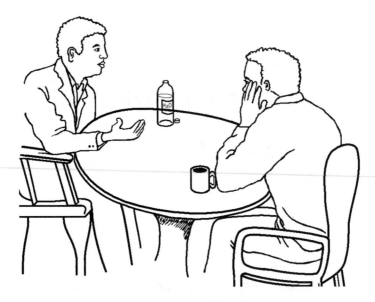

- may order DNA analyses to confirm the mutation.

Based on this information, the counselor can then determine the chances that the parents will pass on a gene with a mutation to their offspring.

Besides informing prospective parents whether they are likely to pass on the gene with a mutation, *the genetic counselor helps after the baby is born by ordering tests that allow precise diagnosis.* Screening for sickle cell is offered in all states, and it is mandatory in most. Screening tests make more effective treatment possible, and inform parents what symptoms they may expect in their child. Genetic counselors often participate in confirming the diagnosis in the infant, determining the risks in future pregnancies, and identifying other family members who may be at risk for having a child with sickle cell disease.

If there is a chance that the couple will pass the sickle cell trait or disease to a baby, the counselor will talk to the parents about the resources they will need to raise a child with sickle cell disease. The counselor will also describe the effect the disease is likely to have on the parents' lives as well as the child's. They may also help the parents understand testing that is available during the pregnancy to determine if the child is affected before birth.

Here Is an Outline of What the Screening Tests May Tell the Counselor and the Parents

Case #	Parent #1	Parent #2	Children*
1	Sickle cell disease Hb SS	Sickle cell disease Hb SS	100% of children -> sickle cell disease Hb SS
2	Sickle cell disease Hb SS	Sickle cell trait Hb AS	50% -> sickle cell trait Hb AS 50% -> sickle cell disease Hb SS
3	Sickle cell disease type SC or Hb SC	Normal Hb AA	50% trait Hb AS 50% trait Hb AC
4	Normal Hb AA	Normal Hb AA	100% normal Hb AA
5	Sickle cell Trait Hb AS	Sickle cell trait Hb AS	25% normal Hb AA 50% trait Hb AS 25% disease Hb SS
6	Sickle cell trait Hb AS	Normal Hb AA	50% trait Hb AS 50% normal Hb AA
7	Sickle cell trait Hb AS	Hemoglobin C trait Hb AC	25% trait Hb AS 25% trait Hb AC 25% normal Hb AA 25% disease Hb SC
8	Sickle cell trait Hb AS	Beta thalassemia trait	25% trait AS 25% beta Thal trait 25% normal Hb AA 25% disease S beta thal

* Percent (%) represents the chances of hemoglobin pattern each child may have with each pregnancy.

FINDING AND WORKING WITH A GENETIC COUNSELOR

You can find a genetic counselor by contacting your local health department as well as state genetic services coordinators. University hospitals are usually good sources of information because they are affiliated with medical schools and usually provide high-quality medical care and research.

Your primary care doctor or specialist can direct you to a nearby university hospital. The local community sickle cell organization may also provide or know of sources for genetic counseling. Other sources of information on genetic counseling resources may be neighbors who are doctors, nurses, or medical technicians, or friends who have already been down this road. You may also contact your state or county's medical society, or any of the organizations listed in Chapter 21, "Resources," for referrals to university hospitals. The National Society of Genetic Counselors' Web site can help you find a counselor at *http://www.nsgc.org*.

THE PARENTS' OPTIONS

A counselor can help determine the odds, but only the parents can decide whether to bring into the world a child who may have the severe symptoms and pain of the disease, and who may not live a full life-span.

Some couples would rather not risk having children who are likely to be born with sickle cell disease. Such a couple has three options:

- avoid pregnancy completely;
- have the baby only when they know, through prenatal tests, that the fetus is perfectly healthy; or
- request preimplantation genetic diagnosis (PGD, for short), which many infertility clinics now offer.

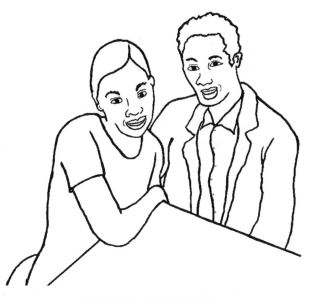

AVOIDING PREGNANCY

Avoiding pregnancy is the simplest and least expensive option. It is also safest to the mother, although a couple may naturally feel emotional pain knowing they can never have their own biological child.

Couples have several ways of avoiding pregnancy:

- Contraceptives, such as condoms or foams, are readily available at the local drug store. Remember that it takes only one incident of unprotected sex to impregnate a woman. Because the choices are difficult once the woman is pregnant, couples should talk frankly with one another about the importance of contraception.
- Another method of avoiding pregnancy is sterilization. The male can undergo a vasectomy, which is the tying of the tubes that allow sperm to move from the testes to the penis. The female may have her fallopian tubes (the organs in which the eggs are fertilized) tied. Neither operation affects sexual performance. Both are usually, but not always, nonreversible.

ABORTING ALL BUT HEALTHY FETUSES

The second option is to have the baby *only* if tests determine that the fetus is healthy. This option may create new obstacles for the couple.

One obstacle is religion. Abortion is prohibited by the Islamic religion as well as by the Roman Catholic Church. Many Protestant churches also discourage or forbid abortion. It is not permitted in Orthodox Judaism, with several exceptions.

Religion aside, many women—and of course many men as well—feel that it is morally wrong to abort the fetus at any stage of the pregnancy.

Legal restrictions on abortion may also pose difficulties. While abortion has been legal in all states for a quarter of a century, many states have recently placed restrictions on it. Ask your legal advisor about the abortion laws in your state.

PREIMPLANTATION GENETIC DIAGNOSIS

The third option for a couple that has decided not to risk having a child born with sickle cell disease is *preimplantation genetic diagnosis* (PGD). PGD is an option for some parents because it doesn't require them to decide to abort the fetus if it will be born with sickle cell disease. This procedure involves taking eggs from the woman's ovary *before* she is pregnant and fertilizing them in a laboratory dish.

When the fertilized eggs begin to divide, one of the cells is taken out for DNA analysis and tested for sickle cell anemia and any other genetic disease. If the embryo is genetically normal, it is implanted into the mother, who completes the pregnancy. If it has the disease, the embryo is discarded.

Infertility clinics would be the best resource for PGD.

PROSPECTS FOR THE FUTURE

Today the genetic counselor's primary role is to:

- provide information about genetic diseases and available resources;
- predict the likelihood of a healthy baby; and
- inform the parents of the available options.

In the future, the counselor might be able to do much more. Researchers are working on gene therapy solutions; however, there are still many difficulties to overcome before this method can be used on humans. (See Chapter 18.)

DETECTION THROUGH PRENATAL TESTS

The prenatal tests that diagnose birth defects, including sickle cell disease, are amniocentesis and chorionic villus sampling:
Amniocentesis is performed (under local anesthesia) by inserting a large needle through the abdomen in order to withdraw a small amount of the amniotic fluid. The sample fluid contains cells from the fetus that can be grown and whose DNA can then be analyzed.

This procedure can be done only in the sixteenth through the eighteenth weeks of pregnancy, and the results take two to three weeks. This means that the woman will be well into the pregnancy before she can be tested and get results. Because the test must be done fairly late, the woman faces some risks from the sampling procedure itself.

Another procedure for prenatal diagnosis is *chorionic villus sampling* (CVS). This can be performed somewhat earlier, at 12 to 14 weeks, and the results can be seen within 48 hours. However, the faster procedure carries 1%–2%

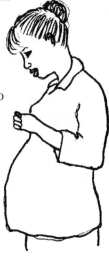

greater risk of miscarriage. Furthermore, the test is less accurate. This means there is a higher possibility that some women, on the basis of this test, might accidentally abort babies who would have been perfectly healthy.

NEWBORN SCREENING

All states in the United States now provide universal newborn screening for hemoglobin problems, including sickle cell disease. If babies can be screened at birth, parents can be alerted to take preventive measures, like providing daily penicillin, a treatment that saves many lives.

If your baby is born in a hospital, blood tests are usually done in the newborn nursery. If you are not sure if your child was tested, have your child retested with the simple blood test called *hemoglobin electrophoresis*.

SUMMING UP

The truths we wrestle with through genetic counseling can be bitter, but the nature of sickle cell disease requires that we think about them:

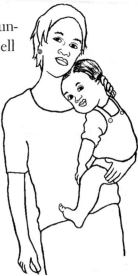

- Under certain conditions, a man and a woman who love one another may be well advised not to have children.
- With all the other problems in your life, it is also important that you know your genetic map. That is the only way you can *decide,* in good conscience, whether to risk passing sickle cell trait and sickle cell disease down to the next generation.

PART TWO

DEVELOPMENTAL ISSUES

CHAPTER EIGHT

Birth to Six Years

The symptoms of sickle cell disease, and its treatment, change over the course of the patient's life. In the next chapters we will talk about these stages of development, beginning with infancy and early childhood.

Let's start with what parents and health care providers need to focused on. First, the clinical issues, period by period.

CLINICAL ISSUES
BIRTH TO 6 MONTHS

- Have the child's hemoglobin electrophoresis done to confirm the sickle cell diagnosis.
- Find a sickle cell clinic, or see a physician with sickle cell experience.
- Learn all you can about sickle cell disease symptoms and prevention.
- Schedule physician clinic examinations once a month, usually when immunizations are due.
- Begin giving the child penicillin, 125 mg liquid by mouth twice a day, at least by two months of age.
- Learn how to recognize fever, how to take temperature, and the importance of penicillin.

- Learn all you can about well baby care.
- Get appropriate immunizations, especially the pneumococcal vaccine Prevnar™.
- If you are grieving about your child having sickle cell disease, share that grief with friends, clergy, or counselors.
- Have your extended family tested for sickle cell, and make a family pedigree.
- Meet with a genetic counselor.

6 MONTHS TO 1 YEAR

- Begin giving the child folic acid (1 mg).
- Learn about nutrition, prevention of complications and accidents, hand-foot syndrome, recognizing illness, and spleen sequestration.
- Schedule clinic visits for every two months.
- Continue all immunizations.
- Join a support group, or talk to other parents with sickle cell disease infants.
- Report concerns and issues to your physician.

1 TO 2 YEARS

- Continue all immunizations.
- Discuss with your doctor pain control, growth/development, and issues related to lifelong disease.
- Schedule clinic visits every three months.
- Each clinic visit should include a physical examination, CBC, and reticulocyte count.
- Get the pneumococcal vaccine, 23 valent, at age two.
- Blood chemistries should be done twice a year.
- Watch for signs of infection, stroke, and increasing anemia.
- Learn the importance of hydration and diet.
- Learn to recognize normal growth and development milestones.

2 TO 6 YEARS

- Increase the penicillin dose to 250 mg twice a day, by mouth, and continue folic acid.
- Continue to learn about normal growth and development milestones, hydration, avoidance of over-dependence, and setting limits.
- Schedule clinic visits every three months.
- Complete all immunizations.
- Learn about pain-management principles.
- Educate school nurses and teachers about sickle cell with handouts, meetings, and letters.

PSYCHOSOCIAL ISSUES

During this period, a child goes through many miraculous changes. He or she will take that first step, begin to talk, and develop a growing sense of self as a social being. For the parents of children with sickle cell disease, these changes bring their own problems. During this period your child will become aware that his or her physical life is different from that of his or her companions. It is not easy to tell a child about an illness that he or she may have for a lifetime. Nor is it easy to cope with a child who is simply fed up with the demands of chronic disease, and sometimes refuses to cooperate.

TALKING WITH YOUR CHILD

Talking with a child about chronic disease should take place only in stages, according to the child's level of understanding at the time. Of course, your child will have questions. So will your other children. The best policy, is to answer your children's questions simply and factually, in terms they can understand. Don't be grim or sad, but don't lie or sugar-coat the truth either. Kids will always see through our lies, however well-intentioned, and a certain amount of precious trust will be lost.

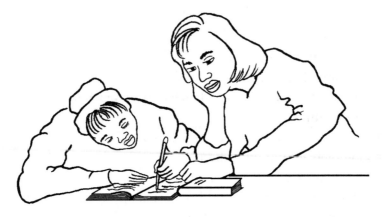

WHAT TO DO WHEN YOUR CHILD ACTS OUT

Like anyone with a chronic disease, your child will sometimes get fed up with taking pills, seeing doctors, and going for blood tests. A child's resistance to treatment can be heart-breaking. It peaks in the preteen and teen years, when some kids not only won't cooperate but deliberately do things that they know can provoke sickle cell crises—like not drinking enough water—in order to manipulate the rest of the family.

At an early age, children learn that when they have a pain episode they get a lot of extra attention and, more often than not, get their way. Sometimes, they may resist treatment, feeling that such resistance gives them power.

The best way to avoid these attention- and power-seeking episodes is to keep the lines of communication with your child open. If you can do that, your child, should he or she choose to act out, can usually be talked back into good sense. But sometimes even a parent's best efforts may fail. That's when family counseling may be helpful.

In general, what the child, or any person suffering a disability, wants to know is what to expect from the disease, and what to expect from the health care system in the way of treatment. The better the child is prepared for the pain and discomfort that the disease, and sometimes the treatment itself, may bring, the better he or she will be able to go along with it.

Your own patience and love will make themselves felt. Trust that. In the bad times, friends, relatives, and counselors can help, as can support groups. Be willing to lean on those who will gladly help you carry the weight.

COMMON MANIFESTATIONS

Knowing what symptoms to expect prepares you to react to them. Here are signs to watch for as your child grows.

BIRTH TO 2 MONTHS

Babies of this age generally have no symptoms of sickle cell disease because they still have enough fetal blood to protect them against the effects of sickle hemoglobin or hemoglobin S.

3 TO 6 MONTHS

Symptoms of sickle cell disease often start at this age, when the baby's fetal hemoglobin is quickly being replaced by adult sickle hemoglobin. The first warning sign in the child is often a painful swelling of the fingers and toes, referred to as *hand-foot syndrome*, or *acute sickle dactylitis*. This is the result of an imbalance between the demand for, and the supply of, blood in these fingers and toes. Rapidly growing bone marrow chokes off its own blood supply by narrowing, or compressing, the blood vessels.

In a baby with sickle cell disease, fever can be caused by a life-threatening infection. Medical care should be obtained immediately. Caregivers should know how to take the child's temperature and diagnose a fever.

Signs of fever in the baby include:

- extreme crankiness;
- incessant crying;

- rapid breathing;
- screaming even when touched or held by family members;
- lack of energy;
- poor appetite; and/or
- decrease in the number of wet diapers (which indicates dehydration).

In the United States and other parts of the world where malaria has been eliminated, the first episode of sickle cell pain is often brought on by bacterial infection. Where malaria is still common, the first episode is typically brought on by malarial infection.

6 MONTHS TO 5 YEARS

For the sickle cell patient, this period of childhood is characterized by:

- a progressive breakdown of the child's red blood cells and subsequent anemia that shows itself in pallor (paleness) of the palms, soles, lips, and eyelids; and
- jaundice, or yellow discoloration of the skin and the whites of the eyes, due to the deposition of bilirubin, a pigment generated from the breakdown of hemoglobin.

COMPLICATIONS

Unfortunately, sickle cell disease can cause any number of secondary complications. Being familiar with them prepares you to cope with them should they develop.

HAND-FOOT SYNDROME

Sickle dactylitis, or hand-foot syndrome, is one of the first complications seen in sickle cell disease, usually occurring between ages six months and two years. One third to one half of patients may experience this complication during early childhood; it is very rare in later life.

Hand-foot syndrome is the result of blocked blood flow and damage to the small bones of the fingers and toes, which causes a rapid, painful expansion of the bone marrow cavity of these small bones. This painful swelling of the back of both hands and feet was the symptom that led to diagnosis before newborn screening became common.

Treatment of hand-foot syndrome includes hydration and pain control with acetaminophen. Bone changes occurring during episodes of dactylitis can be caused by, or mistaken for, osteomyelitis (infection in the bone).

FEVER AND INFECTIONS

Bacterial infections are the most common cause of death in children with sickle cell disease during the first five years of life. Those under three years are at greatest risk for life-threatening infections, but dangerous infections can be seen at any age. The sickle cell patient's decreased ability to fight off overwhelming infection is the result of the spleen not working properly. The spleen is the body's major defense against deadly germs. Serious infections such as blood infections (sepsis), infection surrounding the brain (meningitis), and lung infection (pneumonia) caused by these germs are common and often may be life-threatening.

The bones and joints may also become infected. Infections of the bladder and kidney are more common and may be more severe than in individuals without sickle cell disease. Lives can be saved by detecting these infections early and treating them with the proper antibiotic.

Preventive measures include the following:

- giving daily penicillin at birth until age six;
- giving pneumococcal conjugate and Hemophilus B vaccines, immunization for hepatitis, meningococcus, and influenza, and routine immunization for childhood diseases;
- washing hands after bathroom breaks;

- knowing how to check for fever and learning what to do about it; and
- not eating undercooked meat, poultry, shellfish, eggs, and egg products like mayonnaise, which can allow bacteria to enter the bloodstream from the digestive system.

Be especially careful with warm-weather celebrations like picnics, barbecues, and family reunions, which can lead to steep, rapid climbs in the concentrations of bacteria like Salmonella and Campylobacter in these types of foods because they are not constantly refrigerated. These bacteria do not necessarily make the food taste peculiar. Also, be attentive to washing fruits and vegetables carefully if they're not going to be peeled, as their outsides may harbor some of these same bacteria, as well as pesticide residues. Do not cut or chop any food that will be served raw, such as fruits or vegetables, with knives or chopping boards that have been used with meat, poultry, shellfish, fish, eggs, or egg products without first washing them thoroughly with soap and hot water. Remember that Salmonella is also a common cause of bone infections (osteomyelitis) in folks with sickle cell disease. You might well want to consider adopting a well-balanced vegetarian diet to reduce the risk of contracting some of these common foodborne illnesses.

All sickle cell patients with a fever should consider it an emergency, and consult a doctor immediately.

SPLENIC SEQUESTRATION

The spleen is an organ in the upper-left area of the abdomen, under the lower ribs. The spleen filters out abnormal red blood cells and helps the body's immune system fight infection. Sometimes, in persons with sickle cell disease or other hemoglobinopathies, red blood cells can be trapped in the spleen, a condition known as splenic sequestration. This is similar to bleeding internally because the blood trapped in the spleen cannot circulate to the heart or brain. This condition can range from mild to life-threatening, depending on how much of the body's red blood cells are trapped.

Because splenic sequestration is a sudden trapping of unusually large amounts of blood in the spleen, the spleen enlarges rapidly. The movement of blood from general circulation into the spleen can lead to shock or circulatory collapse.

Patients experiencing this episode may show any of these signs:

- rapid heartbeat (tachycardia);
- shortness of breath;
- dizzines;s
- tiredness and weakness;
- stomach swelling—left upper area (due to the enlarging spleen); and
- fever.

Doctors detect splenic sequestration by feeling for the enlarged spleen and testing for low red blood cell counts. You also can learn how to feel for an enlarged spleen. It only takes some training and practice. Your healthcare provider can teach this to you when you bring in your child for a checkup.

The use of a wooden tongue depressor as a "spleen measuring stick" provides an accurate way of assessing and recording spleen size at home and in the clinic. In small children, one end can be placed on the left nipple and the distance to the spleen tip recorded in ink and dated. In older children, the distance from the ribs to the spleen tip in the left nipple line is recorded. Limits can be set by drawing red lines in ink and instructing the parent to bring the child in for immediate care if the spleen is increased to the line. Parents should check the spleen size on a regular basis and whenever the child appears ill. Names and phone numbers of people who need to be contacted can be written on the back of the spleen stick. Parents should bring the spleen stick with them to every follow-up and emergency visit.

If your child is doing well, then feel for the spleen several times a week just to get practice. You should always feel for an enlarged spleen if your child:

- looks pale, which may be a sign of blood loss. In darker-skinned people, paleness may be easier to detect by looking at the lips, the inner eyelids, and the fingernail beds. Usually these areas are red or dark pink, but if they look light pink or white, then the child is pale.
- seems unusually tired, another sign of a low blood count.
- is unusually cranky or irritable, and perhaps has a headache. When the red blood cell count is very low, oxygen delivery to the brain may be inadequate, causing a headache.
- is sensitive to touch in the upper-left part of the abdomen — the area overlying the spleen.

If you suspect that your child has an enlarged spleen or is displaying any of the above symptoms, take him or her immediately for a medical evaluation. In a child with sickle cell disease, splenic sequestration can be extremely serious, and speedy evaluation and treatment may save his or her life.

Splenic sequestration may happen more than once. To prevent this, your doctor may start you on a monthly blood transfusion program or schedule surgery to remove the spleen, a procedure known as an elective splenectomy.

STROKES:
BLOCKED BLOOD FLOW TO THE BRAIN

Strokes are common in children with sickle syndromes. Strokes may occur in the first year of life, and 80% occur before the age of twenty. There is a very high recurrence rate, approaching 85% in the three years after the first episode. Symptoms of a new or impending stroke include:

- seizures;

- slurred speech;
- fainting; and/or
- weakness and loss of sensation (numb feeling in the face, arms, or legs).

A stroke occurs when blood flow is blocked to a part of the brain by sickled cells or by bleeding from a burst blood vessel. Stroke is an emergency requiring hospital admission, MRI or CT scans, and immediate blood transfusions. Special rehabilitation may be needed with physical and speech therapy to recover skills that may have been damaged.

More commonly, smaller strokes may cause subtle changes in the child's personality or thinking and may leave temporary or permanent function problems. In some strokes, the vessels supplying the brain are blocked for only a short time; this is called a *transient ischemic attack* or TIA. A TIA is a serious warning signal to start preventive strategies with monthly blood transfusions. This monthly treatment keeps the hemoglobin S level at less than 30%. This helps prevent the first major stroke and can also help prevent future strokes if one has occurred.

You cannot stop monthly transfusions once they've started, because stopping them would make a stroke likely to occur. And remember, monthly blood transfusions cause iron overload. They mean exposure to other people's blood, which can build up to a reaction, and it also means exposure to infectious diseases.

Bone marrow transplantation from an HLA-matched brother or sister may offer children who have had strokes the best chance for a more normal life. Children with increased risk for stroke may be detected by transcranial Doppler (TCD) ultrasound screening. (See next section.)

Although "clot busters" are often used in vasoocclusive stroke that is not associated with sickle cell disease, their role in early treatment of strokes in those with sickle cell disease has not yet been tested.

In general, the medical team treats stroke victims by:

- supporting breathing and heart functions;
- preventing bedsores;
- preventing aspiration of food;
- supporting good nutrition;
- avoiding infection; and
- aggressively using physical and occupational therapy to prevent loss of joint flexibility and muscle strength and other rehabilitation for speech, memory, or other issues.

TCD AND STROKE PREVENTION

Sickle cell disease is one of the few conditions associated with childhood stroke, and occurs in 8% to 12% of children with certain types of sickle cell disease: Hb SS and Hb S beta^0 thalassemia. Stroke in these children usually results from a narrowing or closure of arteries supplying blood flow to the brain. Transcranial Doppler ultrasound (TCD) is a device that uses painless sound waves to detect areas of increased blood flow in the blood vessels of the brain. When the blood vessels are narrowed due to sickle cell damage, the blood makes a louder noise as it travels faster through the narrow area. This is like the noise in a water hose when you make the hose bend. When this test detects a constriction, or narrowing, of the blood vessels, there is a greater risk of having a stroke and further testing is necessary.

Studies have shown that transfusions markedly reduce the likelihood of the first stroke in high-risk children with positive TCD results. Annual TCD screening is recommended for all children with sickle cell disease type Hb SS and S beta^0 Thal between the ages of 2 and 16. A listing of centers with approved TCD screening capability can be found on the Sickle Cell Information Center Web site.

ACUTE CHEST PAIN

Children with sickle cell disease may experience chest pain as a result of:

- blocked blood flow to the lungs;
- infectio;
- pneumonia;
- part of the "all over" pain of a pain episode; and/or
- sickling in the ribs.

Acute chest syndrome occurs when there is blocked blood flow to the lungs from infection. The person may have chest pain when he or she breathes in and out, fever, weakness, or a high white blood cell count. This medical emergency is a common cause of hospitalization.

PAIN EVENTS

A pain episode is the most frequent acute symptom of sickle cell disease. While some patients may go for years without an episode, others may have an episode once or twice a month or more. Some of these may be very severe, requiring narcotic painkillers and intravenous fluids.

While some pain crises may occur without an obvious trigger factor, the triggers for most pain crises are:

- fever;
- low oxygen levels;
- *acidosis* (a change in the blood chemistry to the acidic side caused by infection, exhaustion, drug reactions, liver, kidney, or lung problems);
- stress;
- chilly temperatures; and
- dehydration.

These triggers can all lead to sickling of the red blood cells, with clumping of groups of sickled cells and blockage of blood vessels. The resulting low blood flow to the target tissue causes pain.

Pain crises often involve the arms and legs, as well as the head, abdomen, chest, and back, depending upon which blood vessel is being blocked. The pain episode may be extensive, causing severe bone pain and secondary infection of the bone and bone marrow.

A pain episode is commonly treated with liberal amounts of oral and/or intravenous fluids, oral or injectable pain medicines, and treatment of the triggers that caused the pain.

Abdominal organs may be affected during a pain crisis. Repeated damage to the spleen eventually leads to its destruction through a condition called *auto-splenectomy*. The loss of the spleen can in turn increase a person's risk for serious infections. This happens early in life for those with Hb SS, and later in life for those with Hb SC or Hb S beta thalassemia.

Other abdominal organs besides the spleen may be affected during pain crises. The symptoms may resemble the symptoms of appendicitis or gallbladder attacks. In fact, an abdominal pain episode and an abdominal surgical emergency can sometimes happen at the same time.

MORE SEVERE ANEMIA

In sickle cell patients, anemia, or a less than normal number of red blood cells, is lifelong, starting in the first year of life as the fetal hemoglobin level falls. The average red blood cell life span is reduced from a normal 120 days to an average of 10 to 20 days. This causes the bone marrow factory to work overtime in order to make new red blood cells at a faster rate. When red blood cells break apart, the hemoglobin inside is converted to bilirubin, which can make the white part of the eyes look yellow, or jaundiced. In later childhood and early adult life, the excess bilirubin causes gallstones.

A splenic sequestration episode occurs when the sickled red blood cells become trapped in the small blood vessels inside the spleen. This is a cause of anemia (discussed in detail in the Sequestration section).

When the bone marrow factory stops making new red blood cells, it is called an *aplastic episode*. It occurs most commonly during early childhood, but it can occur at any age. The person with this episode has all of the symptoms of having fewer red blood cells, including increasing tiredness, weakness, shortness of breath, dizziness upon standing, and increasing paleness.

Treatment of an aplastic episode starts with a careful decision about whether to give a blood transfusion. (Too rapid a correction of the low hemoglobin can lead to fluid overload and congestive heart failure.) If the cause of the infection is bacterial, antibiotic therapy may be indicated as well.

As we explained earlier, those with sickle cell diseases already have a shortened red blood cell life span. When infection is present, red blood cell destruction (hemolysis) is further sped up.

Treatment for a hemolytic episode is with blood transfusion, fluids, and treatment of any infection.

PREVENTIVE MEASURES
PENICILLIN

Because infections are among the greatest dangers to those with sickle cell disease, all children from birth until age six should be given daily penicillin. The low dose of penicillin is not enough antibiotic to rid the body of an invading infection, but it helps the body to defend itself until you can get the child to a medical facility for more powerful antibiotics. The usual penicillin dose for newborns until age two is 125 mg twice a day as a liquid. At age two, the dose goes up to 250 mg twice a day. This simple low-dose penicillin treatment has saved many patients' lives. Liquid penicillin must be refrigerated and replaced every two weeks if not used.

VACCINATION

Children with sickle cell disease should have all of the immunizations recommended for other children. Immunizations help the body build natural defenses against invading germs and viruses. The new pneumococcal poly valent vaccine named Prevnar™ is a breakthrough that gives protection from birth through the vulnerable early childhood period. Vaccination, plus daily penicillin, will reduce the chance that fatal pneumococcal infection will occur. It is not a guarantee, so parents must be on the watch for signs of infection, mainly fever. Do not continue to give acetaminophen or NSAIDs longer than the recommended time after vaccination. Seek medical care if fever or irritability persists.

INCENTIVE SPIROMETERS

Incentive spirometers, or blow bottles, should be used by the child during any pain episode or event that causes bed rest. The blow bottle is a way to keep the lungs' air sacks open and allow oxygen to get to the red blood cells. Using the blow bottle can help prevent deadly chest syndrome.

BONE MARROW TRANSPLANT

Bone marrow transplantation may be considered if there are dangerous complications like stroke and acute chest syndrome, or frequent pain episodes. The child needs to have an HLA-matched donation from a brother or sister. Successful bone marrow transplant has cured several children worldwide from having sickle cell disease. The procedure has a risk of death in up to 8% of those going through it. The procedure takes several months and costs nearly $300,000. A full description of bone marrow transplant is in the chapter on new treatment and research.

Sickle Immunization Schedule Adapted from the
American Academy of Pediatrics 2010 Recommendations

Birth or First Visit	Hepatitis B Vaccine #1
1 month	Hepatitis B vaccine #2 (or 4 weeks after #1)
2 months	RV, DTaP, IPV, Hib, PCV$_7$
4 months	RV, DTaP, IPV, Hib, PCV$_7$
6 months	DTaP, Hib, PCV, Hepatitis B vaccine #3 (or 6 months after #2)
7 to 11 months	Hib two doses 2 months apart
12 months	PPD, Influenza*, Varicella, PCV$_7$
12 to 14 months	Hib one dose
15 months	MMR Hib Booster if initial 12–15 months
18 months	DTaP, IPV
24 months	Pneumovax®
4 to 6 years	DT, IPV, PPD
5 years	Pneumovax® or Booster Pneumovax®
11 years	Menigococcal conjugate vaccine (MCV$_{-4}$)
12 to 16 years	Td, PPD, MMR booster
16 years	Every Year Influenza*, PPD
Every 10 years—	Td

* Sickle cell at high risk for influenza. See annual recommendations in Morbidity and Mortality Weekly Report . For details and contraindications, see package inserts or recommendations of the American Academy of Pediatrics or National Immunization Program, available at: www.cdc.gov/nip.
DTaP = Diphtheria, acellular Pertussis vaccine, Tetanus toxoid
Hib = Haemophilus B Conjugate vaccine
PPD = Tuberculin test
IPV = Inactivated Polio Vaccine
MMR = Measles, Mumps, Rubella
Pneumovax = 23-valent pneumococcal vaccine, only given once if the first dose is administered after age five
PCV$_7$ = Heptavalant conjugate pneumococcal vaccine
Td = Tetanus, Diphtheria—Adult dosage
Vaccination, penicillin prophylaxis, and prompt attention to fever can prevent serious pneumococcal infections. Conjugate vaccine against S. pneumonia for infants is available—Prevnar—and should be given according to the recommended schedule along with pneumovax (see health care maintenance). Adults should receive S. pneumoniae immunization with polysaccharide vaccine once every five years and yearly influenza immunization. S.B.E. prophylaxis should be given if heart murmurs may be caused by valve pathology or if hip or other prostheses are in place.

Heptavalent Pneumococcal Conjugated Vaccine (PCV7) in Children with SCD Schedule Up to the Age of 5 Years (adapted from the AAP recommendations 2000)

Age of First PCV7 Dose	PCV7 Primary Series	PCV7 Booster Dose	Pneumovax®
2 to 6 months	3 doses 6–8 weeks apart	1 dose 12 months	2 doses 2 years* & 5 years
7 to 11 months	3 doses 6–8 weeks apart	1 dose 24 months	2 doses 2 years* & 5 years
12 to 23 months	3 doses 6–8 weeks apart	1 dose 24 months*	2 doses 2 years* & 5 years
24 months to 4 years, no Pneumovax	2 doses 6–8 weeks apart	none	2 doses 2 years* & 5 years
24 months to 4 years, had Pneumovax	2 doses 6–8 weeks apart	none 5 years*	1 dose

*   6–8 weeks after last PCV$_7$

Suggested Heptavalent Pneumococcal Conjugated Vaccine (PCV7) in Children with SCD Schedule 5 Years and Older

Age of First PCV7 Dose	PCV7 Primary Series	PCV7 Booster Dose	Pneumovax®
5 years & older no Pneumovax	1 dose	none	1 dose*
5 years & older had Pneumovax	1 dose*	none	

*   6–8 weeks after last PCV$_7$
Some authorities recommend revaccination every 5 years with pneumovax patients at risk, practice varies among sickle cell clinics.

CHAPTER NINE

Six to Twelve Years

By age six, the routines and procedures described in the previous chapter will be established. But some new symptoms will appear, and some of the old ones will become more pronounced. You will have new tasks to do, such as monitoring your child's medical condition and helping your child keep up good preventive practices.

Also during this period, your child will start school, and you will want to have a clear understanding with his or her teachers and other school staff members about the special requirements your child may have.

In this chapter we will talk about these new issues.

CLINICAL ISSUES

- Talk with your child's doctor about stopping penicillin.
- Schedule clinic visits every four to six months.
- Start scheduling full eye examinations every year.
- Identify gallstones with an ultrasound test.
- Have your child screened for hearing loss and pulmonary function (breathing).
- Have urine screening for protein, a sign that the kidneys may be having difficulty.

PSYCHOSOCIAL AND PARENTING ISSUES

- Stress academic achievement, prevention of complications, and health maintenance.
- Begin sex education.
- Keep track of your child's psycho-social development.
- Be prepared for delayed puberty.
- Set limits for behavior.
- Encourage good school performance.
- Be sure you and your child keep doctors' appointments.
- Do not let sickle cell rule the house.
- Spend quality time together doing fun and memorable activities.
- Allow normal activities, keeping in mind FARMS prevention.
- Try not to favor the child with sickle cell disease over other brothers and sisters, giving all quality time. There may be episodes of hospitalization during which the normal daily routine is disrupted. Let the other children know what is going on, and let them be involved as much as possible.

"SICK ROLE"

Give your child care and compassion, both when the child is well and pain free as well as when ill and in pain, with equal amounts for all of your children. Avoid making a big fuss and "rewarding" the child in times of pain and illness. Some children, and adults, who are rewarded with attention only when they are ill or in pain develop a "sick role," using pain in order to gain attention. Your aim should be to motivate the child to get better and to continue with the daily routines of school, friends, and activities.

CAMP

Many sickle cell foundations and clinics sponsor a sickle cell camp during the summer for children six to twelve years old.

These camps allow the children to have fun with other kids with sickle cell disease, in a medically supervised environment. These camps usually have adult sickle cell patients as counselors to help mentor the younger patients.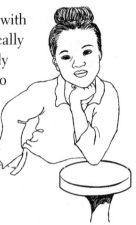

Check with the sickle cell community group and clinic near you to see if a camp is offered.

AGE-SPECIFIC SYMPTOMS

- The inability to concentrate urine will become more obvious. Affected children will urinate more often, and persistent bed wetting *(enuresis)* may occur. These problems understandably lead to difficulties in the child's socialization. Normal activities like camp, sleepovers, school trips, and even sitting through classes become potentially embarrassing for the child. Bed wetting may become a source of conflict between the parent and the child if the parents do not understand the cause.

- More severe anemia may develop. This is caused by early red blood cell breakdown (hemolysis). This breakdown releases hemoglobin into the blood stream, where it is converted to bilirubin. Bilirubin causes the white part of the eye to turn yellow (jaundice).

- The spleen may be regarded as a filter for broken red blood cells, removing them from the circulation. As a result of removing the damaged cells from the blood stream of those with sickle cell disease, the spleen enlarges. Occasionally, this organ experiences pooling of large volumes of blood; this is called a *sequestration episode*. These two processes combine to produce enlargement of the spleen.

- Your child will have an increased need for calories and energy to build new red blood cells and repair damaged tissue.

- Abnormal development of the jaw and/or breast bone occurs in some individuals. The bone marrow expands as it tries to accommodate the need for increased red blood cell production. The primary expansion sites include the jaws and the breast bone. Prominence of the forehead (known as *frontal bossing*), and protrusion of the jaw (known as *prognathism*) are among the abnormal bony symptoms of some people with sickle cell disease. Because the jaw protrudes, dental abnormalities and gum disease may occur more often in these children.
- Any decreased performance in school work may signal that your child is having silent strokes. Have your doctor order magnetic resonance imaging (MRI) of the brain and psychological testing.

COMPLICATIONS

New secondary problems can develop in children with sickle cell disease during this period.

GALLSTONES

Gallstones can form in the gallbladder, which holds bile, a substance made from bilirubin, the by-product of hemoglobin recycling. Bile helps your body digest fatty foods. Because of the increased red cell hemolysis in sickle cell disease, bilirubin production is increased, and this causes gallstones to form in the gallbladder.

Gallstones can cause the gallbladder to become plugged and swollen. This causes pain in the upper-right area of the stomach, nausea, and vomiting. These symptoms can happen especially after eating fatty or fried foods.

If necessary, the gallbladder can be surgically removed.

DELAYED GROWTH

Children with sickle cell may weigh less than others of the same age, though this varies from child to child. Older children and adolescents with sickle cell disease, on the average, are shorter than their peers, but this difference disappears in adulthood. Puberty may come later in both males and females with sickle cell disease. Factors contributing to the delay include the low red blood cell count, and the type of sickle cell disease. In general, it is better for the individual with sickle cell disease to not be overweight, so good nutrition and not overeating should be stressed.

Treatment for delayed growth includes good general nutrition, vitamins, increased calories, and, on the psychological side, reassurance that normal maturation will occur.

PRIAPISM

Priapism is the painful erection of the penis caused by sickling red blood cells blocking blood flow out of the penis. Priapism usually occurs between the ages of 5 and 35. It often occurs as a severe, long episode requiring hospitalization and follows multiple episodes of short duration, termed "stuttering." Episodes may come from infection, having sexual intercourse, masturbation, or normal night-time erections. Onset in the early morning, awakening the patient, is common.

Treatment for priapism includes pain relief, medication that opens closed blood vessels, hydration, blood transfusion, and surgery. Impotence is a long-term consequence of repeated episodes in one-third to one-half of the cases.

KIDNEY PROBLEMS: BED WETTING, PROTEIN

The kidney has just the right conditions—low oxygen, high salt concentration, and high acid concentration—to cause red cells to sickle. The kidney is the main filter of the blood, saving or releasing water, salts, and waste products. If early damage impairs the kidney's ability to retain water, it can let too much go—even when the the body is dehydrated.

When the kidney releases too much water, children may wet the bed at night and may need frequent bathroom breaks. This is important to discuss with teachers and caregivers. To help control the bed-wetting problem, use an alarm that sounds when dampness is detected. These are available at most drug stores. Encourage your child to stop drinking fluids one hour before going to bed.

Over time, damage to the kidney filters can cause protein to leak into the urine. This is the first sign that more damage is occurring. A special urine test for protein, with data collected over 24 hours, can help predict the level of damage that may occur. There is research underway to test preventive medications that may slow this kidney damage.

PREVENTIVE MEASURES

- Again, the best strategy for prevention is FARMS, as outlined in the previous chapter.
- Be sure that, when your child exercises or works outdoors, he or she wears the proper clothing for the season, carries a water bottle, and drinks plenty of water. He or she must take frequent rest and water breaks.
- Your child should avoid swimming pools that are too cold or hot tubs that are too hot. Even when swimming in a warm pool, he or she should dry off immediately when getting out of the water to prevent chilling that may cause a pain episode.
- Your child should avoid emotional stress by pacing projects and work, and by avoiding situations likely to be upsetting.
- Parents and child should belong to a support group. This will often be, according to your beliefs, a church or faith-based group that can offer spiritual and emotional support.
- Transcranial Doppler ultrasound testing should continue annually until age 16 for children with Hb SS and Hb S beta^0

thalassemia. See the previous chapter for further information on this test as a means of stroke prevention.

HYDROXYUREA

The effectiveness and safety of hydroxyurea was established in the late 1990s for adults with sickle cell disease. Hydroxyurea is now accepted therapy for pediatric sickle cell patients. Nonetheless, the treatment has been relatively uncommon among pediatric patients. It is more common among teenagers, and most common among adults.

While there is still much to be learned about hydroxyurea therapy for sickle cell patients, we know this:

- Hydroxyurea treatment seems to improve pain; reduce anemia; and prevent acute chest syndrome, priapism, and abnormal red blood cell stickiness to the blood vessel wall (endothelium).
- Hydroxyurea decreases the frequency of pain episodes, though it may not completely eliminate them.
- Small studies have shown no impact of hydroxyurea on sickle cell damage to the spleen and, perhaps, no impact in avascular necrosis of bones such as the hip and shoulder joint.
- Hydroxyurea prolongs life.

New information about side effects and episode-reduction benefits will come out during the next several years, but, at the moment, the side effects for children on hydroxyurea appear to be the same as the effects for adult patients. These are some of the potential side effects of long-term hydroxyurea therapy.

Common side effects:

- Mild nausea or upset stomach. Most patients have this only for the first few weeks at a certain dose, then the nausea goes away. Sometimes nausea is less troublesome if the hydroxyurea is taken at bedtime.

- Suppression of blood cell production. Mild suppression is an intended side effect of hydroxyurea, but hydroxyurea dosing needs to be carefully adjusted and blood cell counts monitored every two to four weeks to make sure that the suppression does not become severe. Hydroxyurea may suppress the white blood cells too much, leading to increased chances of infection; suppress platelet counts too much, leading to increased chances of bleeding; or suppress red blood cell counts too much, leading to worse anemia, with fatigue and problems for heart and lung function.

Possible side effects:

- thinning of hair;
- darkening of skin and nails; and
- abnormal sperm counts or sperm movement.

Rare side effects:

- decreased kidney or liver function;
- dizziness;
- changes in mood or thought; and
- excess chances of intracranial bleeding unrelated to platelet counts.

All of these effects are expected to be reversible when the hydroxyurea is stopped. Generally, the medication can then be adjusted to a lower dose.

LEUKEMIA

Some people on hydroxyurea for other blood disorders seem to have an increased rate of developing leukemia (cancer of white blood cells). However, it is possible that sickle cell disease by itself—and not the hydroxyurea treatment—predisposed those people to leukemia. Studies in groups of sickle cell patients on hydroxyurea have not revealed increased DNA damage that would make us suspicious of leukemia development.

BIRTH DEFECTS

So far, the handful of babies born to mothers on hydroxyurea for sickle cell have not had birth defects. But worry about the possibility of birth defects leads most doctors to give hydroxyurea only when individuals in the reproductive ages are on good contraception. Males or females on hydroxyurea should abstain from sex or use excellent contraception. It is recommended that hydroxyurea be stopped before conceiving a baby to help avoid the chance of birth defects.

GROWTH AND DEVELOPMENT PROBLEMS

Some people have worried that hydroxyurea treatment will slow the growth or development of children with sickle cell disease. A few years of tracking several dozen children has not revealed growth and development problems so far, but longer experience is needed.

HYDROXYUREA THERAPY IN A NUTSHELL

Hydroxyurea therapy for a child with sickle cell disease has many possible benefits, several known risks, and several potential long-term side effects. The full details of the levels of these risks will not be known until we have done more research into sickle cell hydroxyurea treatment.

We strongly recommend individual discussions with your child's hematologist about the risks and benefits for you or your child. At Grady Hospital, we generally have two or three sessions in order to:

• review the child's medical history and present condition;
• discuss individualized risks and benefits;

- provide reading material on these risks and benefits;
- draw a panel of baseline lab tests (blood counts, vitamin B_{12} and folate levels, kidney function and liver function, check for hepatitis and HIV infection, test for pregnancy); and
- check a brain MRI scan for any signs of stroke or abnormal blood vessels that might increase the chances of bleeding in the head.

You need to have a doctor who will follow your child very closely for blood counts and monitor for hydroxyurea-related or other sickle cell problems.

ALTERNATIVE TREATMENTS

Besides managing the complications of sickle cell disease as they occur, the only other current alternatives to hydroxyurea therapy are:

- regular transfusions; and
- bone marrow transplantation (You will find a detailed review of bone marrow transplantation in Chapter 16.).

Both of these alternatives have major risks as well as major benefits. Talk with your doctor about the risk/benefit balance for you or your child.

Still other treatments for sickle cell disease are in the research pipeline, but none is likely to be available outside of a clinical research trial for a couple of years.

GUIDE FOR TEACHERS

It is a good idea to meet with your child's teachers and find out what they know about sickle cell disease. If there is a school nurse, let him or her know about your child. Most sickle cell clinics have a handout to give teachers. You can also help educate your teachers. Here is a sample guide you can modify to your special needs.

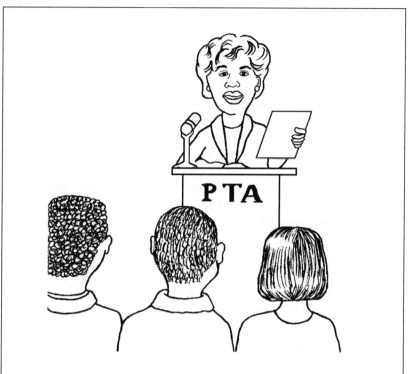

Sample Classroom Guide

- Sickle cell patients may be absent because of severe pain episodes caused by the blockage of blood flow to body organs or bones. These episodes may require treatment in a hospital setting. Make-up work for students should be provided to keep the student current with assignments. A hospital- or home-based teacher may be required for prolonged complications.
- Pain episodes may be prevented by allowing persons with sickle cell disease to keep well hydrated with water. Let them keep a water bottle with them or allow frequent water breaks. They will require frequent bathroom breaks also, because their kidneys cannot retain water as well as normal kidneys.
- Pain episodes may also be prevented by not allowing the individual to become over-heated or exposed to cold temperatures.
- Because of their anemia, individuals with sickle cell may tire before others. Rest periods may be appropriate.
- Encourage gym and sports participation, but, because of anemia, persons with sickle cell may tire before others. Allow them to stop and take breaks without undue attention.

(continued)

Sample Classroom Guide (continued)

- Sickle cell disease is a lifelong illness that may have various effects that can impair academic performance. These should be identified and addressed, as they would for any child. Academic performance is especially important now that life expectancy for those with sickle cell has increased dramatically. Those with sickle cell, like anyone, can become professionals like doctors, engineers, and lawyers.
- Sickle cell patients may have a yellow tint to their eyes because of the increased bilirubin for red cell breakdown, but, this is not usually a liver problem. They also may have a shorter stature and delayed puberty because of the anemia.
- Students with sickle cell should be treated as normally as possible, with an awareness that they may have intermittent episodes of pain, infection, or fatigue that can be treated and sometimes prevented through adequate water intake and by, avoiding temperature extremes and overdoing it.
- Learn about sickle cell, and understand the challenges that students with this disease must face.
- Have a plan of action with the individual to do what you can to keep him or her productive and complication free.

Medical attention is needed when any of the following occur:
- fever;
- headache;
- chest pain;
- abdominal pain; or
- numbness or weakness.

A mild pain episode may be managed with increased fluid intake and a non-narcotic pain pill like ibuprofen or acetaminophen.

Your school can launch a sickle cell awareness program by encouraging activities like these:

- Invite a speaker from your local sickle cell foundation or clinic to educate the entire class or staff about sickle cell.
- Become involved in public awareness events like walks, fun runs, kids' camp, and fund-raisers.
- Encourage blood donations and blood drives in your community. Many with sickle cell need transfusions to prevent childhood strokes and other complications.
- Support sickle cell research to provide new treatments.
- Encourage sickle cell patients to be the best they can be.

Disabled School Children and the Law

An important law to consider is the Individuals with Disabilities Act (IDEA), PL 101-476, which states the rights of children with disabilities, and of their parents. A basic part of the law is the right of parents to help decide about their child's education. IDEA says, "States must provide a free appropriate public education to all students (ages 3–21) who are disabled. Children must by assessed for their disabilities, strengths, and needs."

Another important law to keep in mind is PL 93-112, the Rehabilitation Act, Section 504, which was designed to end discrimination on the basis of a physical or mental disability in any program getting federal financial aid—as well as public schools. Some children with health problems may not need, or be eligible, for services under IDEA, but they may need special help or modifications under Section 504. Some examples of modifications may include a shortened school day/week, special equipment, and modified academic coursework.

Hospital/Homebound Services: This is a plan for children in kindergarten through 12th grade who have missed school at least 10 days due to illness, and who may miss more. A teacher is sent by the school system to the home for at least three hours a week.

What Parents Can Do

- Become active in your child's school. Get to know the teacher and school staff, and maintain open communication.
- Be very clear about what you want for your child. Tell teachers about your child's illness. Let teachers know how to meet your child's school needs. Tell them what you know about your child's physical problems. For example, your child may have a hard time carrying books or have problems keeping up in gym when sickle cell problems occur. Also tell the school staff to be alert to the signs of sickle cell difficulties, such as fatigue, fever, and jaundice.
- Keep in mind that, if your child needs to be in the hospital, he or she may use the hospital's school program. You can help by bringing your child's homework to the hospital's schoolteachers so that your child may continue to receive school credit. Being a part of the hospital's school program also helps to decrease the pressure on your child by helping him or her keep up with schoolmates.
- Ask school staff members to share their observations of your child with you.
- Keep a good relationship with the school staff.
- Attend all meetings that are held, such as parent/teacher conferences and Individualized Education Plan (IEP) meetings. Bring a friend or family member with you who knows your child. Take notes, and don't be afraid to ask for time to think about a certain decision.
- Keep track of your child's progress. Is the plan you agreed on working? Do any changes need to be made? Check in with the teacher often to seen how things are going. Keep a notebook to give and receive information.
- It is important for your to understand your child's illness. The disease may cause depression, withdrawal, sleeping too much or not enough, acting out, or changes in eating patterns in your child. If any of these things happen, it would help to speak to a mental health professional for your child and possibly for the entire family. It is important to seek help to deal with the pressures involved with a child with sickle cell disease.

(continued)

What Parents Can Do (continued)

- Be aware of the needs of any other children you may have. They may feel anxious, angry, or depressed. A sibling may feel guilty because he or she is healthy. They may feel lonely and withdrawn because the child with sickle cell disease is getting a lot of attention, especially during periods of pain crisis or when in the hospital.
- Sickle cell disease my affect learning in some children. If there is concern about a child's ability to learn, discuss this with your physician as soon as possible. If a child has had a history of strokes, it may be necessary for him or her to receive psychological testing to determine ability to learn.
- Children with sickle cell disease may be absent a lot due to clinic visits, pain crises, or other health problems. Make sure classwork and homework assignments are available to you to keep the student from falling behind. If your child is in the hospital, communicate with the hospital's teachers and give them his or her classwork. If necessary, arrange tutoring for your student.
- Keep in mind that children with sickle cell disease tire more easily that other children. *This is important for the physical education teacher to understand.* These children should be given the time to rest when needed. Physical activity is an important part of good health, so it is best to include them even if they are hesitant. If you prefer that your child be excused from any activity, permission should be granted.

CHAPTER TEN

The Teen Years:
Thirteen to Eighteen

HEIDY'S STORY

For as long as I can remember I have longed to be normal, and sometimes that longing made my life even harder than it was already. I was ashamed to be ill, and sometimes angry that pain episodes and other medical problems kept me from living what to me seemed the free and easy lives of my friends.

But when I was ten, in the hospital for treatment for one of my many pain episodes, something clicked. I sat up in bed and told myself I'd never feel sorry for myself again.

The way I remember coming to that insight and resolution was this. I'd been hospitalized more than 100 times for pain episodes. I understood what caused the pain, but that didn't make the trips to the emergency room any easier. I knew the treatment. Strong drugs like morphine and Demerol and fluid given to me intravenously.

I hated the trips to the emergency room, even though without them I couldn't get rid of the pain. Sometimes the pain was okay, but sometimes I felt as if I were about to die. Month after month, I'd have one of these crises, and I'd pray to God for an answer to the question I never stopped asking: "Why me?"

Sometimes when I was a child I'd ignore the limits the doctors had warned me about. I'd swim in the school pool, even though I'd sometimes get sick afterwards because the water was too cold. I was trying very hard to kid myself. I actually believed for a while that if I didn't think of myself as being sick I wouldn't be, so I ignored many warnings and tried hard to hide my sickness from friends and family.

That went on for years, and during that time I wasn't doing very well as a patient. When I was older and a little more open to reason, my doctors told me that I would be able to deal with sickle cell disease only if I learned about it. So I did learn.

As I got older I understood that sometimes I had to deal with doctors and nurses who didn't know much about sickle cell disease. I made it my business to educate them by telling them patiently about the illness and about what I needed to make my symptoms more manageable. I began to follow the research, and to know about the people and clinics searching for a cure. To sum it all up, as a child I was afraid to tell the truth about who I really was. I was afraid even to know that truth myself. Now I accept it, and I let other people know because I realize that sickle cell disease is part of me.

Today I can honestly say that, in a way, sickle cell has become a blessing. It has made me stronger by making me come to terms with myself. I know I'm one of the lucky ones. There are some people out there with this disease who lack the help they need. I have a loving and understanding family. Even though they can not feel my pain, they are with me every step of the way. As for friends, they come and go, but there are some I have had since childhood who cry every time they see me in pain. I am thankful for them.

My quest for normalcy has faded into a devotion to aid, as much as I can, those with my disease. I am now at the beginning of a new quest to find a cure for my disease.

COMMON MANIFESTATIONS

As Heidy could tell you, each stage of maturation brings new problems and the need for new solutions. Adolescence can be hard on anyone, but it is especially hard on people with sickle cell disease. A broad range of physical ailments can, and does, occur.

AUTO-SPLENECTOMY

The previously enlarged spleen begins to shrink from tissue death (*infarction*) caused by inadequate blood supply. As a result of this shrinkage, the spleen may disappear entirely by the end of adolescence. (Doctors call this *auto-splenectomy*—literally, the body performing a *splenectomy*, on itself.) While the teenager can live without a spleen, it does have important immune functions; without it, the patient will probably experience more infections. These infections, in turn, increase the risk of more crises.

PRIAPISM

In males with sickle cell diseases, priapism, or painful prolonged erections of the penis, may occur as a result of sickled cells blocking the outflow of blood from the penis. Repeated episodes of priapism can, unfortunately, lead to erectile dysfunction and permanent impotence. Clinical trials are beginning to study better ways to treat priapism. Although none have been studied in clinical trials, medications used to prevent priapism include hydroxyurea, pseudoephedrine, etilefrine, tenocetaline, and sildenafil.

CHRONIC LEG ULCERS

Chronic ulcers may form, especially on or near the inner side of the ankles. They result from blockage of the blood supply to the skin by sickled red blood cells and other material. The ulcers generally appear pale, with a yellowish tinge. More details about leg ulcers are in the next chapter.

CHRONIC BONE INFECTIONS

Chronic bone infections with chronically discharging openings are all too common. These bone infections (known as osteomyelitis) are difficult to cure. Sometimes they require months of intravenous and/or oral antibiotic therapy, often combined with localized surgery. X-rays, bone scans, and gallium scans (a type of imaging) are helpful in suspected cases of osteomyeitis. Definitive diagnosis usually requires biopsy, with culture, to prove the infection and determine which antibiotics will work the best.

DELAYED PUBERTY

Puberty in children with sickle cell disease is sometimes delayed, as it is in children with other debilitating, chronic illnesses. For girls, the onset of the first menstrual period (or *menarche)* and breast development may both be late. In boys, the testicles remain small longer, and body hair growth may be delayed. Puberty will eventually come.

EMOTIONAL PROBLEMS

Emotional problems result from trying to deal with the overwhelming range of problems—the fatigue, bouts of acute illness, pain, fear of death, and social isolation. Depression is common and can be treated by professional counselors and antidepressant medications. School grades can fall. Drug abuse may occur as a way of coping with physical and emotional pain.

PREVENTIVE MEASURES

Patients and parents will already be familiar with the best ways to prevent pain—a set of guidelines known as FARMS. See Chapter 2 for a discussion of these guidelines.

NO SMOKING, NO ALCOHOL, NO DRUGS

Smoking robs the red blood cells of oxygen. Alcohol dehydrates the body and can damage the liver over time. Alcohol can also make the blood more acidic, and this can cause sickling. Finally, alcohol impairs judgment and can lead to mistakes.

Illegal drugs like cocaine can cause episodes of pain. They kill people without sickle cell and are even more dangerous in those with it.

BIRTH CONTROL OPTIONS—SEXUALITY

Parents should counsel teens about the benefits of abstinence and monogamous relationships. But if the teen is sexually active, prevention against HIV and sexually transmitted diseases is critical.

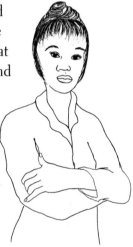

- The combination of a latex condom and spermicidal foam provides safe, effective contraception and *is the only method* that may reduce the transmission of AIDS and other sexually transmitted diseases. The condom should be put on before any penetration.
- Oral contraception is probably the most effective method and is probably safe if progesterone preparations are used. But it presents a higher risk of complications if a teenager is a smoker, is overweight or obese, or has a clotting disorder, such as lupus. It is generally used after a woman has had one or more children.
- The IUD is also effective, though with this form of contraception there is increased risk of infection.
- Diaphragms are usually less effective, but may be satisfactory if combined with a spermicidal preparation.
- Progestin-based prevention by pill or depo injection preparations is also effective. But please note that progestin-only-based contraception may result in unpredictable bleeding. It may also increase LDL or "bad" cholesterol and decrease HDL, the "good" cholesterol. It may also increase triglycerides and blood pressure.

- Even with the most careful precautions, a sexually active teen may become a mother or a father, so it is vital that your child consider the potential for passing sickle cell disease or trait on to his or her own child. If he or she is involved with a partner, strongly urge the couple to undergo genetic counseling *before* becoming intimate.

Remember that sickle cell diseases are 100% preventable!

Caution: *It is critically important to know that oral contraception, IUDs, diaphragms, or progesterone will NOT protect you against HIV/AIDs.*

CLINICAL ISSUES

- Discuss sexual development and related issues with your child.
- Assist your child in progressing to independence, stressing self-management, coping skills, and academic achievement.
- Discuss with your child birth control, prevention of complications, learning physical limits, sexually transmitted disease, and substance abuse.
- Provide peer support by encouraging support group contact and activities.
- Discuss realistic job and career goals and and education beyond high school.
- Schedule clinic visits every four to six months.
- Teens should have a screening test to detect protein in the urine. This may be the first warning about kidney damage.
- Teens should have a screening test called an echocardiogram to detect high blood pressure in the lungs (pulmonary hypertension).
- Immunization against human papilloma virus is recommended for girls, to prevent cervical cancer.

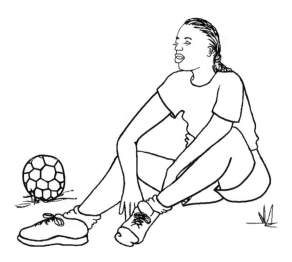

PSYCHOSOCIAL ISSUES FOR TEENS

Teens should be counseled about the serious dangers facing all teens. However, teens with sickle cell disease are at higher risk of injury or death from guns, auto accidents, suicide, drugs, and alcohol than from their disease. Encourage seat belt use, avoiding alcohol, and avoiding those with guns and street drugs. Risky sexual behavior can lead to unwanted pregnancies, HIV, and other sexually transmitted diseases. It is important to spend time with teens affirming and supporting them. Supportive friends and parents can be positive influences.

Explore the symptoms of depression or drug abuse, including sleep disturbances, eating disorders, lack of interest in favorite activities, and withdrawal from friends and family. Ask about suicidal thoughts and plans. These should be taken very seriously and professional help sought immediately if such plans are revealed.

PUBERTY

Puberty may be delayed by two to three years in those with sickle cell disease. Teens and parents should be assured that puberty will occur. With the onset of puberty come emotional highs and lows.

Self-esteem may suffer when one's peers are growing and developing secondary sex characteristics, and you are doing so at a much slower rate.

TRANSITION TO ADULT HEALTHCARE TEAM

It is important to make the transition from pediatric services to adult caregivers over a period of time. The treatment philosophy is quite different in a children's hospital from that of an adult in-patient ward. Take time to get to know the adult doctors, nurses, and social workers. Learn about all of the adult services available. Some centers offer teen clinics to meet the special needs of adolescents. One major problem in the United States is finding an adult doctor who will care for sickle cell adults. Start by looking for a hematologist with training in sickle cell. The next best physician would be an internist or family practitioner with an interest in sickle cell disease.

Teens can get ready for this transition starting years before the switch to adult caregivers.*

Practice talking to the doctors and nurses about your health history and health care while still accompanied by your family. Practice getting ready for an appointment so that you get the most out of it:

1. Do you have any new problems or questions? Write them down before the visit so you can make sure to bring them up.
2. Collect your insurance information and other medical papers.
3. Collect your medications, and know which might need a new prescription.
4. Be ready to take notes about new information.

*Adapted from the American Society of Hematology—make the most of your appointment.

MEDICAL HISTORY KNOWLEDGE OUTLINE

You know that people will ask you the same questions over and over again about your medical history. People with sickle cell disease can have complicated medical histories, so a smart healthcare provider will want to learn more about you before trying to start taking care of you. You might as well get ready by having the answers before your medical visit. Some families keep a "health passport." It might help a teen get familiar with his or her medical history to make a notebook with key medical information.

1. Do you know what type of sickle cell disease (hemoglobin SS, SC, S beta thal) you have?
2. Do you know your baseline hemoglobin level?
3. Do you know your baseline pulse ox level?
4. Do you know all of your medication names and doses?
5. Do you know all of your drug allergies?
6. Do you know all of the surgeries that you have had?
7. Do you know if you have received any blood transfusions?
8. Do you know whether you developed antibodies because of past blood transfusions?
9. Have you ever had a transfusion reaction?
10. When you have sickle cell pain, how do you treat your pain? What activities ease your pain? What medications usually help you?
11. Have you had any sickle cell problems like: stroke, acute chest syndrome, splenic sequestration, acute chest syndrome, or sepsis?

CHAPTER ELEVEN

Young Adulthood:
Nineteen to Twenty-Five

MELISSA'S STORY

I was three years old when I was diagnosed with sickle cell disease. Living a few miles from the beach, it was just another day when my parents and I went to the ocean. It became a day unlike any other, though, when that night I was restless and ill, and nothing seemed to calm me.

In the morning my parents took me to our family doctor, and he arranged for me to have some tests, which over a series of weeks led to more tests. At one point, the doctors thought I had leukemia. My physician noticed my spleen was enlarged, and that, combined with the suggestion from my aunt, a nurse, to look into being tested for sickle cell, sparked my diagnosis. The test showed that this was just what I had.

Both of my parents had emigrated from Jamaica to the United States, and, although the disease is common in Jamaica, unfortunately neither of them had even heard of it. They didn't know that they each carried a gene for altered hemoglobin, which left them untouched but had a drastic effect on my own genetic make-up. The hemoglobin portion of my red blood cells (the part that carries oxygen to all of my body parts) was changed so that sometimes it caused my normal blood cells to sickle. My parents were told that I had the SC variant. Though my parents were from Jamaica, the same scenario happens every day here in the United States due to lack of information and lack of access to that information.

My parents were aware I had a disease, of course, but they tried not to emphasize that I might be different from anyone else. I also learned lessons the hard way, by sometimes denying my difference. For example, the kids in our fifth grade gym class were expected to run a mile to complete an end-of-the-year physical aptitude test. Instead of telling my instructor that I was tired, I pushed myself to exhaustion. I completed the run, but I missed the rest of the school year. The strains that triggered episodes weren't always physical. During my junior year in college, I was so stressed out about a test that I ended up in the ER. I was hospitalized only twice during my adolescence and young adult years. The fact is that the disease, in whatever form, does not affect everybody in the same way or with the same severity. Learning about the sickle cell trait was very important to me, because that trait had so much to do with who I am.

In Jamaica, about 10% of the population has the sickle cell trait, but, on other islands, the frequency varies from 7% in Barbados to as high as 13% to 14% in Dominica and St. Lucia. This compares to about 8% in the black American population, and frequencies of 20% to 30% in black populations of West Africa and of some populations in Saudi Arabia, India, Greece, and Italy. So it's important to find out if you carry the sickle cell gene by getting a simple and painless blood test called hemoglobin electrophoresis. Getting tested is easy. Tests can be arranged by your general practitioner or at your local sickle cell center or foundation. Soon, nearly everyone will be screened at birth. Newborn screening is mandatory. Even today most states will require newborn screening.

When I was three, there wasn't much going on in sickle cell research or treatments. Twenty-odd years later, the outlook for someone like me who has the disease has improved tremendously. In the past, survival beyond the age of 30 was unlikely. Now it's common for many of us with the disease to live to old age.

There's still plenty of work to be done. In my community, and many others, access to medical care can be difficult for a lot of people, but improvements are occurring as people learn more and more about how to find the medical help they need. I've made this my life's work. I received a master's in public health with health education—the focus of both my studies and vision for the improved quality of life for those whom sickle cell disease affects.

Where there's ignorance, there's myth, and myths surround sickle cell disease. Health education is about dispelling health myths. It's important to remember:

- Sickle cell disease is not contagious; it is a genetic disorder you receive from birth.
- It is not cancer.
- The mind is not affected.
- It is not just a "black" disease but affects Hispanics and people of Asian and Mediterranean origin as well.
- It is not "bad blood" or a family curse.

Sickle cell is a disease that exists just as any other except in a way unlike any other. In its uniqueness, it offers challenges to both those who treat it and those who live with it. It is a disease that has molded my life and made me who I am and hope to be.

COMMON MANIFESTATIONS
LEG ULCERS

Leg ulcers cause chronic disability in 10% to 15% of older children and young adults with sickle cell anemia. Leg ulcers in those with sickle cell diseases start as a result of localized tissue death in the skin, which in turn is caused by clogging of small blood vessels with sickled red blood cells and blood clots.

Treatment includes the following:

- Medication. Many individuals with leg ulcers are deficient in zinc, and zinc is required for white blood cells to fight infection and for wound healing. Most individuals with leg ulcers should take supplemental zinc pills.
- Good nutrition.

- Preventing swelling in the legs through elevation and by wearing supportive stockings is one of the most important treatment and prevention methods.
- Removing dead tissue. This speeds healing and prevents infection. It is done using hydrophilic dressings.
- Using a zinc-impregnated bandage or unna boot twice a week.
- A bioengineered temporary skin substitute called Apligraft™.
- Using wet/dry dressings.
- Bed rest and leg elevation.
- Grafting. When leg ulcers cannot be healed by any other means, surgical skin grafting may need to be performed.
- Blood transfusion therapy.

It's always a good idea to exclude additional causes of ulcers, such as diabetes, peripheral arterial disease, and venous stasis, all of which have specific treatments.

Many ulcers may be prevented with good skin and foot care. If your skin tends toward being dry and ashy, try using a good skin-lubricating lotion twice a day. Some excellent ones include Eucerin™, LacHydrin™, and Carmol™. Don't go around barefoot at home, in the yard, or at the beach. Splinters, bits of sharp metal, broken glass, or broken shells could be lurking there ready to cut your skin and start the ulcer process. Avoid insect bites from mosquitoes, chiggers, and fleas. Always inspect your legs, ankles, and feet for areas that are painful and/or discolored when you get up in the morning and before you go to bed at night. Use a handheld mirror if necessary. Show any such areas to your doctor or podiatrist (foot doctor) as soon as possible. Avoid buying unsuitable shoes because they look "hot." Early care may help to prevent an ulcer from progressing and possibly becoming infected.

AVASCULAR NECROSIS OF THE HIPS AND SHOULDERS

The round part of the hip bone and shoulder bone each have one artery supplying blood flow to keep the bone alive and healthy.

This artery can be blocked by sickled red blood cells. If this happens it could cause the round end of the bone to die. This condition, avascular necrosis, is most common in Hb SC and S beta thalassemia type sickle cell disease.

In a patient with avascular necrosis, the affected area begins to collapse, making the round ball shape turn rough and jagged. This causes pain when walking or moving the leg at the hip joint and in the arm in the shoulder joint.

The first line of treatment is to use daily arthritis medications that are safe (see the chronic pain treatment section). But the long-range objective is to prevent further joint destruction by taking weight off the hip by using a cane or crutch, and by limiting walking. The shoulder is rested as much as possible. A physical therapist can help teach you how to exercise to maintain flexibility and strength without damaging the joint further.

Once the pain level becomes too high and can't be controlled with medications or physical limits, a visit to the orthopedic surgeon for a consultation about a joint replacement should be scheduled. The surgeon may recommend an artificial hip or shoulder joint. Highly advanced new materials make these joints last much longer than previous models of artificial joints. Many doctors have changed their recommendations about joint replacement in young adults with sickle cell disease, and suggest artificial joints at earlier ages than before. Ask your doctor to discuss how long an artificial joint might last in your situation, how much pain relief and function you might have, and how long you would need to devote to physical therapy rehabilitation exercise after a joint replacement. Studies show that hip replacements do not last as long in young, active individuals and that many will have to be replaced because of wear and loosening after an average of 7 to 10 years.

The risks of joint replacement include postoperative complications, joint infection, and joint failure. The surgeon should work with your sickle cell doctor to ensure the safest possible surgery, with a preoperative blood transfusion to raise your hemoglobin to 10, good hydration, and incentive spirometry (blow bottles) after surgery. After a hip joint replacement, rehabilitation exercise for several months with coaching by physical therapists will strengthen your muscles and make the joint stable again.

EYE PROBLEMS

Blocked blood flow in the small blood vessels in the back of the eye causes the eye to make new, weaker, blood vessels to bypass the blocked ones. These new blood vessels are thinner and tend to break open, causing bleeding into the clear eye fluid. This can also cause the retina, the seeing part of the eye, to detach. The result can be reduced vision or blindness.

Patients with Hb SC disease, and perhaps sickle thalassemias, are at increased risk for these eye complications. Yearly eye examinations by an eye doctor, with appropriate use of laser surgery, if necessary, may reduce the severity of these complications.

People with diabetes may develop a retinal disease that is quite similar to sickle cell retinopathy. Measures that have been successful in preventing the development and progression of diabetic retinopathy include reducing elevated blood pressure to not more than 130/80 and use of ACE inhibitors whether or not the blood pressure is high. We do not yet have any studies to prove whether these measures are effective for people with or at risk for sickle cell retinopathy. People with diabetic retinopathy are also told to avoid constipation and straining, drink plenty of water, and eat plenty of fiber. If would seen logical that these measures would be the same for people with sickle cell disease.

REPRODUCTION AND PREGNANCY

CAN PEOPLE WITH SICKLE CELL DISEASE HAVE CHILDREN?

Yes, but planning is key. Sickle cell disease affects your ability to conceive a baby and to carry a pregnancy to full term. Sickle cell disease has life implications that should be factored into the decision to have children. Raising children is hard work, making emotional and financial demands that may be doubly challenging because of sickle cell disease.

Remember that sickle cell is an inherited disease. Your choice of a mate will directly affect the chances that your child will also have sickle cell disease. If your spouse has sickle trait, then there is a 50% chance that your child will have sickle cell disease. If your spouse has normal hemoglobin, then none of your children will have sickle cell disease, but some may have sickle trait. If your spouse has a trait for beta thalassemia or some other hemoglobin abnormality, there may be a 25% to 50% chance that your child will have sickle cell disease. (See chapter 6 for more about genetics.)

ARE MEN WITH SICKLE CELL FERTILE?

Yes, but men with sickle cell disease may have a few issues that affect reproduction.

Priapism can cause severe penile pain when it happens, and also leave scarring inside the penis. Repeated episodes of priapism can lead to impotence—inability to have a normal erection of the penis. One of the reasons that an episode of priapism should be treated promptly is to relieve pain, but another reason is to avoid impotence. (See chapter 10 for more about priapism.)

Sperm counts and sperm motility may not be normal in men with sickle cell disease. Sperm might also be affected by hydroxyurea, and seem to recover when hydroxyurea is stopped.

Though highly discouraged, children have been conceived by men taking hydroxyurea. Yet the long-term effects of hydroxyurea on reproductive success in males are not known. Regardless, men should not plan to father children while taking hydroxyurea, because of the risk of birth defects. (See chapter 17 for more about hydroxyurea.)

ARE WOMEN WITH SICKLE CELL FERTILE?

Yes, but women with sickle cell disease may be affected by several issues that affect reproduction.

For some women, menstrual periods can trigger sickle cell pain. Hormonal control (such as Depo-ProveraTM) to stop menstrual periods also prevents pregnancy. If you come off the hormonal control in order to get pregnant, sickle cell pain episodes may recur. (See chapter 10 for more about menstrual cycles.)

For some women with avascular necrosis of the hip joints, intercourse in certain positions may be very painful to the hip.

So far, no birth defects have been seen in the women with sickle cell who became pregnant while taking hydroxyurea, but some had miscarriages. Furthermore, it is strongly recommended that you do not conceive children while taking hydroxyurea because this medication causes birth defects in laboratory animal testing. Women should discuss child-bearing plans with their hematologist and plan to stop hydroxyurea at least six to eight weeks before becoming pregnant. (See chapter 17 for more about hydroxyurea.)

WHAT ABOUT INFERTILITY TREATMENTS?

Infertility specialists are widely available, but infertility treatment is rarely covered by medical insurance in the United States. The treatment package would probably include preimplantation genetic diagnosis (PGD), which is described on pages 163 and 164. The rate of successful pregnancy is 50% or less, and can result in twins or triplets with premature birth.

Adoption is an option. Adopting a baby can be easier on the body than going through pregnancy, although certainly the adoption process can cause emotional stress.

Some people with sickle cell disease choose not to have children.

HOW IS PREGNANCY AFFECTED BY SICKLE CELL DISEASE?

Pregnancy is hard on any woman's body. Good prenatal care is very important for every pregnant woman and for her baby. This is particularly crucial for a pregnant woman with sickle cell disease.

The increased blood flow and nutrition for the baby in her womb can be a big strain for the heart and lungs of a woman with sickle cell disease. "Morning sickness" can cause anybody to become dehydrated, but dehydration comes even more quickly for a woman whose kidneys are affected by sickle cell disease. For these reasons, pregnancy may be associated with worsening of sickle cell disease, including sickle cell vaso-occlusive pain.

The placenta of a woman with sickle cell might be damaged by sickled blood cells, often causing the baby to be smaller than average. The risk of obstetric problems is especially high for mothers with sickle cell anemia (sickle cell disease SS). These may lead to the baby being born prematurely.

Management of pregnancy in the patient with a sickle cell syndrome requires coordinated care by obstetricians and hematologists knowledgeable in the disease. Although complications have gone down over the last 20 years, there are still some increased risks for both mother and child. With careful management, there is no reason that women with sickle syndromes cannot have children.

All sickle cell patients should receive accurate information at puberty and periodically throughout their reproductive lives about the risks of pregnancy, genetic transmission of sickle syndromes, methods of contraception, prenatal diagnosis, prevention of sexually transmitted disease, and the increased responsibility of raising children.

All pregnant patients should be under the care of an obstetrician with interest and expertise in managing pregnancy in sickle syndrome patients. The primary care physician and hematologist should also be involved as members of the management team.

Most pregnant patients should be on folic acid, prenatal vitamins, and standard iron supplementation unless iron overload is present. Follow-up visits are usually scheduled every two weeks, with weekly visits when necessary for complications, and during the last four to six weeks of the pregnancy.

IS HAVING THE BABY THE HARDEST PART?

Perhaps not. Any parent can tell you that raising a child is tremendously hard work, even with the deep joy in being a parent. Caring for a newborn baby means sleeplessness for weeks, and patiently figuring the needs of a helpless creature who can't talk. Caring for a pre-schooler means keeping watchful eyes on a fast-moving explorer who can't wait to taste, pull on, or climb everything within reach. Caring for a school-aged child means infinite patience with infinite questions: "Why?" Caring for a teenager means wisdom to know when to set limits consistently, when to show affection and encouragement, and when to simply listen and let go. And all of this requires the self-control to be a role model for the child watching how you do things.

All of this is challenging for any parent, but can be doubly challenging for a parent living with an unpredictable health condition like sickle cell disease. It will be triply challenging if your child also has sickle cell disease (see chapters 3 and 8–12). Many parents will plan to live close to family and friends, so that this support system can help with children when they themselves are sick or too tired. Many people wait until they are financially stable before having children. Some choose not to have children.

CAN OUR FETUS BE TESTED FOR SICKLE CELL DISEASE? WHAT STEPS ARE POSSIBLE IF WE FIND OUR UNBORN CHILD HAS SICKLE CELL DISEASE?

Prenatal diagnosis can allow you to find out whether the fetus is affected by sickle cell disease. Probes or needles can be inserted into the placenta for chorionic villus sampling, which can be done early in pregnancy (between 9.5 and 12.5 weeks gestation), but this procedure is somewhat risky. The other prenatal diagnosis technique is amniocentesis (sampling the fluid sac around the baby), which can be done from about 14 weeks gestation to about 20 weeks gestation.

If sickle cell disease is present, you would have a head start on planning a treatment strategy for your child. You can save the cord blood from your child with a private cord blood bank, in preparation for possible gene therapy when it becomes available someday in the future. Be advised that private cord blood banking can cost a thousand dollars or more.

You will have the option to terminate the pregnancy. Yet, for many people, life begins at conception, and the destruction of a fetus is the same as destruction of an individual.

WHAT IS PREIMPLANTATION GENETIC DIAGNOSIS?

It is possible to ensure that a pregnancy will produce a baby free from sickle cell disease. The preimplantation genetic diagnosis (PGD) process starts with "in vitro fertilization" by a doctor specializing in infertility treatment. Medication stimulates a woman's ovaries to produce eggs. The eggs are collected from the mother. The father gives a semen sample. The eggs and sperm are combined in a laboratory. The fertilized eggs each grow over the next three days to an eight-cell embryo. A single cell is removed from each embryo using small instruments. The DNA from each cell is collected and copied through a process known as polymerase chain reaction (PCR). The DNA sequence code is checked with molecular analysis to see which hemoglobin genes are present in each embryo. Embryos that are free of sickle cell can then be transferred into the mother, where they should implant in the womb and be carried as a pregnancy.

There are several concerns about preimplantation genetic diagnosis. For many people, life begins at conception, and the destruction of embryos—even only eight cells—is the same as destruction of an individual. The PGD process usually results in a number of discarded embryos. Some labs give the option to save these embryos for research. PGD is expensive and time-consuming, and may not be covered by health insurance in the United States. Transferring multiple embryos into the mother can result in multiple pregnancies (twins, triplets, or more). This can make pregnancy and child-raising more challenging. Multiple pregnancies are also more likely to result in premature birth.

HOW DO THE DIFFERENT ANTI-SICKLING THERAPIES AFFECT REPRODUCTION?

The anti-sickling therapies currently available can be very effective in fighting sickle cell disease, but they have different side effects. Part of your doctor's role is to discuss with you and your family both the benefits of the anti-sickling treatment and the risks of these side effects in your specific situation. Some of these side effects will affect reproduction. General comments are included here to help you start these discussions with your doctor about your specific situation.

Bone marrow or cord blood transplantation: Transplantation of these stem cells can cure sickle cell disease (see chapter 16). Many of the treatments that prepare the body to accept the transplanted cells have a side effect of infertility for males and females. This infertility risk is especially high for the myeloablative transplants, when the goal of the preparative treatment is to wipe out the marrow that produces sickled red blood cells. Newer experimental transplant preparative treatments may have lower risk of infertility. Males can try sperm banking before the transplant, but the sperm may also have low function due to sickle cell. It is important to remember that the sperm or eggs after transplantation would still carry the genes for sickle cell disease, not the genes of the marrow donor. The risk of having a child with sickle cell disease could be as high as 50%, depending on the hemoglobin genes of your mate. Discuss the risks of infertility when you meet with transplant doctors.

Hydroxyurea: Hydroxyurea can make severe sickle cell disease milder in many ways, and can greatly improve quality of life. Hydroxyurea causes birth defects in lab rodents. Birth defects have not been seen in people after hydroxyurea, but people on hydroxyurea must plan to avoid conceiving children while taking this treatment. Use contraception or abstinence while taking hydroxyurea. Discuss a strategy with your doctor for stopping hydroxyurea if you are planning a child.

Chronic blood transfusion: Monthly transfusions of normal red blood cells can greatly reduce the risks of major sickle cell complications such as stroke and acute chest syndrome. Chronic transfusion often causes iron overload, which can be reduced with daily use of iron chelation medicines such as ExJadeTM, DesferalTM, or deferiprone. If iron overload is not managed properly, it can cause hormonal problems that lead to infertility.

Gene therapy: Gene therapy is just barely becoming available, and there are many risks to consider for this highly experimental therapy. It is important to remember that your sperm or eggs are not the target of gene therapy, and these would still carry the genes for sickle cell disease. Depending on the hemoglobin genes of your mate, the risk of having a child with sickle cell disease could be as high as 50%.

PREVENTIVE MEASURES

In this age group, the FARMS include:

F—Fluids. Drink 8–10 glasses of water a day, and take daily folate, 1mg. Folic acid may help produce more new red blood cells, as well as help blood flow through smaller arteries.

A—Air—Avoid altitudes, smoking, and asthma.

R—Rest when you need to, and don't overdo physical activity.

M—Medications like hydroxyurea may be the best preventive.

S—Situations to avoid: temperature extremes, alcohol, illegal drugs, and tobacco.

CLINICAL ISSUES

- Schedule clinic visits for a history, physical, and CBC every two to six months. A reticulocyte count, and urinalysis should be done at each visit. Get blood chemistries, an eye exam, and a PPD skin test once a year. Screen for gallstones and aseptic necrosis if symptoms occur.
- Keep immunizations up to date, and get an annual flu vaccination.
- Learn all about your sickle disease, pain management, prevention of complications, response to emergencies, and avoiding substance abuse.
- Learn the importance of knowing your limits, hydration, diet, and dental care.
- Ask your provider about disease variability, prognosis, and prospects for future therapy.
- Seek psychosocial support when needed.
- Learn how to do breast or testicle self-examination.

PSYCHOSOCIAL ISSUES

Young adulthood brings new challenges to everyone, and, as always, the challenges will be especially strong for people with sickle cell disease. Three of the new challenges are career choice, raising one's own family, and knowing how to accept and even seek the support of others.

CAREER CHOICES

You'll want to avoid jobs that could make your sickle cell disease worse. These tend to be outdoor jobs with exposure to temperature fluctuations, or manual labor that can cause fatigue and increased sickling. Standing for long periods may cause pain in the hips and knees in areas with blocked blood flow and bone damage. It also may lead to leg ulcers or make them harder to cure.

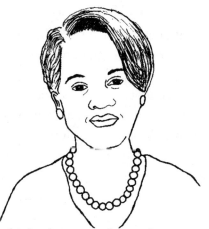

We recommend jobs that are indoors, that are not manual, that have good health insurance benefits, and that are enjoyable. We encourage patients to work hard in school and try to go to college or vocational school. If you choose outdoor work, try to always dress appropriately for the weather—and, if possible, live in an area with mostly moderate year-round temperatures.

It is good to work for an employer that understands sickle cell disease and knows that you may sometimes have to miss work because of pain events or other complications. A letter from your doctor with information we have outlined in this book is a good first start.

FAMILY ISSUES

Many people with sickle cell disease choose to live near parents, or brothers and sisters, who can help them when they need transportation, child sitting, help with household chores, and support when complications or severe pain episodes occur. Often, for the family, this is a continuation of a support system long developed. This can provide important support; however, it is important that the adult becomes able to live an independent lifestyle and develop friends and other support networks.

PEER SUPPORT

A successful patient's network will reach beyond the family to other patients, with whom one can offer and receive support and ideas, encourage and be encouraged, help raise community awareness, and advocate for excellent care in the local health care facilities. Monthly meetings at a local home, a meeting room at the library, or the hospital can help keep all informed about the latest news in the community. Communicate with newsletters, phone chains, e-mail, and even Web sites.

CHAPTER TWELVE

Adulthood:
Twenty-Six to Forty

MICHELLE'S STORY

My name is Michelle Rodriguez. I was born in Brooklyn, N.Y., and I am 31 years old. I was born with sickle cell disease. My parents both had the sickle cell trait, though they didn't suffer from the disease. But they did have trouble with diabetes, heart disease, and high blood pressure that ran in both their families.

I don't remember much about how sickle cell struck me in early childhood, but when I was ten my mother told me that I had stayed in the hospital for two months after I was born while the doctors gave me blood transfusions and other kinds of IV treatment.

As a young child I often had sickle cell attacks, and these attacks got worse as I got older. I did what I could with folic acid.

I didn't do very well. My pain was often terrible and I grew weaker. My schooling was interrupted and almost ended by the disease. In junior high school, for instance, I missed two to three months of school each year.

I tried hard to keep my life normal. I got through junior high by going to summer school for an extra semester. I was lucky to have a loving mother who taught me never to give up.

By the time I got to high school, the attacks got less frequent and less severe. I got through my freshman year very well. Then, in the beginning of my sophomore year, I got pregnant. As bad as this can be for any young girl, it was especially bad for me. During my pregnancy, I was in and out of the hospital all the time. I suffered severe joint pains from an infection the doctors couldn't pinpoint.

When it came time for the delivery of the child, I was in crisis. I was suffering such severe joint pains and labor pains at the same time that I was never moved to the delivery room. Hooked to an IV and monitoring machines, torn by the double sets of pain that ran through me, I continued this terrible labor until, finally, the doctors had to deliver the baby by Caesarian section.

I first saw my baby in the nursery, and I wanted to cry. She weighed only two pounds and five ounces, and it broke my heart to see this little infant already hooked to so many machines. I didn't think she'd live.

I'm happy to say that Dominique *did* live. Maybe she inherited that same courage my mother had taught me. I went on to graduate from high school. My sickle cell attacks became much rarer and less severe after my pregnancy. But, shortly after I graduated, I had to have surgery, and when I was recovering the sickle cell attacks grew worse, and I was in and out of the hospital again.

Much of my suffering is behind me, and finally I can say proudly that I have learned to live with sickle cell disease.

Michelle continues to pursue her degree at New York's famous Fashion Institute of Technology, with occasional semesters off, not due to her own illness but to care for family members with other illnesses.

Domenique attends a university in Maryland on a scholarship, like her mom.

COMMON MANIFESTATIONS

BONE PAIN

At this age, more prolonged and constant pain can be seen with bone infarction, sickle arthritis, and aseptic necrosis of the hip bone or shoulder. With chronic pain, the safest non-steroidal anti-inflammatory medications should be given. Hydroxyurea can be discussed with your doctor. Trans-cutaneous electrical nerve stimulation (TENS) units, relaxation techniques, and occupational and physical therapy approaches may be useful in reducing pain and maintaining a functional lifestyle. Education and support are often required to prevent addiction to the drugs that may be used to control the pain.

KIDNEY PROBLEMS

Kidney damage starts very early and progresses throughout life. With advancing age, protein in the urine and kidney damage may occur. All patients should be screened for protein in the urine annually, beginning at age six. The blood pressure medication enalapril has been shown to reduce protein in the urine. If the kidneys stops working, poisons are not filtered out of the blood and you can become very ill.

The next step is dialysis—running your blood through a kidney machine or peritoneal dialysis. Peritoneal dialysis involves putting a filtering solution in the abdomen, letting it stay for awhile to remove the body's poisons, then draining the solution. This form of dialysis can be done at home three to four times a week by the individual or family members. Individuals with sickle cell disease and kidney failure can benefit from kidney transplantation, and this treatment is available in a number of academic centers.

The kidney makes a hormone named erythropoietin that causes the bone marrow to make more red blood cells. When the kidney is damaged, erythropoietin levels may drop, and the bone marrow slows down red blood cell production. This makes the anemia situation worse. This can be treated by giving replacement erythoropoietin (Aranesp™, Procrit™, Epogen™) as a weekly or monthly injection. Hydroxyurea treatment is sometimes combined with erythropoietin to make the red blood cells last longer and improve the anemia.

Those with kidney problems should not take NSAIDs for pain or any other medication, including over-the-counter treatments, without consulting their doctor.

Lung problems

Pneumonias, acute chest syndrome (caused by red cell sickling in lung blood vessels), and fat from bone marrow blockage, are acute complications seen with increased frequency in patients with sickle syndromes. They are sometimes hard to diagnose because signs of chest pain, cough, fever, pulmonary infiltrates, and severe hypoxia are common to all. Reactive airway disease (asthma) is less common in adults than children, but it seems to be more prevalent in patients with sickle cell disease.

Treatment for lung problems involves careful monitoring of hemoglobin and blood gasses, oxygen for hypoxia, IV hydration, pain treatment, and antibiotics. An exchange transfusion may be necessary in episodes with severe hypoxia, rapid progression, or diffuse pulmonary involvement.

Chest syndrome may be prevented by the use of incentive spirometry in all hospitalized patients. Older patients may develop pulmonary fibrosis, chronic restrictive lung disease, pulmonary hypertension, and cor pulmonale. If the oxygen level is always low, then home oxygen may be prescribed to aid breathing.

Hydroxyurea is proven to be useful in preventing repeated episodes of acute chest syndrome. Good asthma care and yearly influenza vaccinations can also help to prevent acute chest syndrome.

PULMONARY HYPERTENSION

Pulmonary hypertension, or increased blood pressure in the blood vessels carrying blood from the heart to the lungs, is a common complication in adults with sickle cell disease. If untreated, it can cause early death. The causes of pulmonary hypertension are multiple, including red blood cell breakdown (hemolysis), low levels of nitric oxide in circulation, chronic low oxygen levels, blood clots, and repeated blood-flow blockage with sickled red cells. It can be diagnosed with a Doppler echocardiogram. Treatment includes the use of nifedipine (a calcium-channel blocker), intravenous epoprostenol, inhaled nitric oxide (NO), and exchange blood transfusions.

PREVENTIVE MEASURES

In addition to normal FARMS prevention, men and women of this age should participate in cancer screening, including mammograms and PAP smears for women, and prostate screening in males. Now that life expectancy is increasing significantly, older sickle patients need to undergo all of the healthcare screenings that are recommended with the general population of their ages.

PSYCHOSOCIAL ISSUES

Most studies have shown that individuals with sickle cell disease do a very good job of coping with their disease and are well adjusted. Chronic pain, missing work, family pressures, depression, insomnia, and anxiety are the most common social issues in this age group. These can lead to further stress, anxiety, and depression. A professional counselor, social worker, clergy member, or psychiatrist can be a great benefit in managing them. There are medications that help depression and help treat chronic pain at the same time. A psychiatrist or your primary care doctor can prescribe these medications. (See chapter 15 for more information.)

PEER SUPPORT

Meeting with other adults with sickle cell disease can help you relieve stress, share resources, and provide coping ideas for the pressures of life. The fellowship of other sickle cell patients can help build self-esteem and improve hope. Invite special speakers to address issues common to all. Get involved; volunteer to be a role model for younger patients.

CHAPTER THIRTEEN

Adults over Forty

INGRID'S STORY

My name is Ingrid Whittaker-Ware, Esq. I was born in 1962 to Raphael and Muriel Whittaker, and was the fourth of five children. I was raised on the sunny island of Jamaica and emigrated to Atlanta, Georgia, in 1980.

I was diagnosed with sickle cell disease (SS) at eleven months old. Although I had signs of jaundice from birth, the doctors did not properly diagnose my disease until I was having an uncontrolled fever and crying more than usual for an eleven month old. I am the only one of my siblings to be born with the disease. Both of my parents have the sickle trait, as do one brother and my little sister.

My parents taught me as a child the value and empowerment of knowledge and determination. Once, when I was having a pain episode, I cried and begged my parents to send me to school. I wanted this so badly that they let me go. That same day, during the lunch hour, I was hit in the head by a stray stone thrown by someone on the playground. The teachers wanted to call my parents right away, but I begged them not to, because I feared my parents would take me home and keep me out of school for several days until I was completely well.

At that time, being in school helped to lift my spirits and take my mind off being more physically challenged than my peers.

I was blessed to have had the expert and compassionate care of Drs. Elaine Reid and Graham Serjeant. To them both I owe a debt of gratitude for the care they provided me while I was growing up. Truly, I have been blessed from the time I was born. When I was diagnosed with sickle cell disease, the doctors did not expect me to live past my sixth birthday. In fact, at first I was diagnosed as having leukemia, and it was not until further testing that the doctors came up with the diagnosis of sickle cell disease.

Despite the gloomy predictions from the doctors, the good Lord is the author of my life and had other plans for me. So, He has always placed me in the care of the very best doctors in the area of sickle cell disease and research. Dr. Reid watched over me the only two times I was hospitalized as a child. The first of those two times I was not expected to live because of the seriousness of the infection. I was very young then and do not remember much about that hospitalization, but I do remember being placed in an oxygen tent and the grim expressions of the medical staff and my parents. I survived then as I am surviving now. Dr. Serjeant cared for me through adolescence into adulthood, and it was he who first taught me to protect my legs from insect bites and injuries in an effort to minimize leg ulcers.

I attended Spelman College and graduated with a double major in three and a half years. At Spelman I majored in political science and economics with a minor in international relations. I graduated *magna cum laude*. Life at Spelman was fun. My professors inspired and challenged me to reach for the stars and further instilled in me the conviction that knowledge is power. For the most part, I stayed out of trouble with sickle cell disease at Spelman, although there were stressful times, what with the pressure of exams and the like. I viewed that type of stress as a positive challenge and managed never to have a serious pain episode for which I had to be hospitalized. I tried my best to take care of myself, by hydrating myself constantly, and follow the healthy practices I learned early in life, which were reinforced by the staff at the Grady Sickle Cell Center.

I had several leg ulcers, and one bout with what was suspected to be osteomyelitis, while I was at Spelman. I remember my mother waking me up early one morning and asking why I was moaning. I told her that I was not moaning, but then immediately felt the pain in my ankle. This was the first time I was given a mild narcotic medication (Tylenol 3™) to help control the pain. I could not do my usual activities that summer, which included working at a summer job. However, I refused to let the summer be an entire loss and decided to take a course in calligraphy. I am still able to write calligraphy today and sometimes get requests from family members to do a special piece for them. At Spelman, I also took time for piano lessons again, which I hadn't done since I was a child. Playing music, particularly the piano, often helped me relax and reduced my stress.

At Spelman, I won the prestigious Thomas Watson Fellowship. This fellowship gave me the chance to travel to Venezuela and extensively in Europe, in the quest of being a "better world citizen." On returning from my travels, in 1985, I enrolled in Columbia University School of Law in New York City. I graduated from Columbia and returned to Atlanta to work as an attorney for the federal government, where I have been for the last thirteen years.

Whether I travel on business or for pleasure, I always take care to properly hydrate myself before, during, and after flying and have never encountered any major sickle cell – related problems due to air pressure. The air does sometimes become a little dry, but I counter that by breathing into a cup with a few drops of water or a few slices of lemon. A flight attendant taught me that trick while I was on one of the long flights from the United States to Venezuela, when the dry air had become uncomfortable to breathe.

During my life's journey, as I have grown older, I have had many challenges. However, I have also had God's protection and His many blessings. Some of my challenges from sickle cell disease have included recurrent and painful leg ulcers and one aplastic crisis. The aplastic crisis racked my body with so much pain that I can only describe it as feeling like I had been hit by a runaway freight train. This aplastic episode was also accompanied by high fevers in excess of 105 degrees. I remember awaking from a feverish sleep to see my husband shivering with cold as he sat in the room with me. The doctors had severely lowered the room temperature to try to bring my body temperature down. I also have frequent pain episodes (for which, thankfully, I usually do not have to be hospitalized), mild retinopathy, and frequent blood transfusions (a fairly recent development). In addition, I had gallbladder disease and a heart attack before age forty. I have also had other illnesses that were not initially sickle cell related, but became so when sickle-related complications developed.

Despite the bleak outlook and shortened life expectancy predicted by doctors when I was first diagnosed with the disease, I am here to tell my story almost four decades later. I have also been blessed with a very supportive family, including a mother and father who had faith that their first daughter would survive and did everything in their power to ensure that I did. Their efforts included making sure they learned as much as they could about the disease and then passing that knowledge on to me so that I could, in turn, take care of myself. My parents maintained appropriate communications with my doctors while I was a child so that I could get proper and immediate treatment when necessary, and to ensure that I had a proper diet and nutrition. They also provided a comfortable, positive, and stable environment in which I could grow up. My three brothers, sister, and extended family and friends have also always been very supportive of me.

Today, I am married to Willie J. Ware Jr., my caring and supportive husband, who stands guard at my bedside each time I am ill. He hovers over me like a mother hen and gets on my case about taking care of myself as much as, or worse than, my mother does. I am also the proud mother of the cutest and most charming three-year-old toddler, William, who came into our family by adoption. I am fulfilled by having the joy and comfort of knowing that I am loved and cared about by not only my husband and son, but by my extended family and friends as well.

To my comrades in arms who live with the disease, I challenge you to:

- develop your spiritual life and ask for God's continued blessings, because—even when the doctors and everyone else give up hope—He is the only one who can bring you through the many trials that you face;
- adopt a positive attitude and know that with God's help you can do anything you put your mind to—so believe in yourself;
- believe that knowledge is indeed power and educate yourself as much as you can about your disease and your body and take all the steps necessary to stay healthy and positive, including maintaining proper contacts with your health care providers and maintaining a healthy diet; and
- continue to have faith and hope that a cure to this disease will be found soon, and do whatever you can to contribute to that cause.

To caregivers, family, and friends, I say thank you—and continue to keep the faith. Keep yourself and your loved ones encouraged. The more you learn about the disease, the more you can help your loved ones and educate others in the fight against sickle cell disease. To health care professionals, again I say thank you. I also challenge you to continue to provide care in a compassionate fashion, treating your patients with the respect and dignity you would accord anyone who comes across your path. You never know—you could be entertaining a future lawyer, doctor, or influential person. Encourage your patients to live as full and productive a life as possible.

COMMON MANIFESTATIONS
MENOPAUSE

There are no reported research articles about menopause in sickle cell patients. At the same time, we have seen clinically that women have more pain events and complications during this time period. Estrogen replacement may or may not be beneficial. Water loss during hot flashes requires additional water intake. Hormone replacement, using Premarin™ (conjugated urinary horse estrogens) or Prempro™ (the same estrogens combined with the synthetic progestin, medroxyprogesterone acetate), has been shown to be associated with an increased risk of stroke, heart attack, and breast cancer and a reduced risk of hip fracture and colon cancer. The study concluded that, for most women, the risks of long-term therapy outweigh the benefits. This study, the WHI, has been widely criticized for its methods, most particularly the age of the women at the time treatment was started [mostly over 60, which may be too old to obtain the cardiovascular benefits] and the particular choice of estrogen and progestin. Nevertheless, most major medical societies have incorporated this study's findings and recommend that, if hormone replacement therapy is to be used, it should be for as short a time and at as low a dose as possible to reduce or eliminate menopausal symptoms.

There are theoretical reasons why, what is called bioidentical hormone replacement therapy, may be safer and more advantageous, but the jury is still out on this one and probably will be for some time.

Several approaches offer alternatives to hormone replacement in menopause.

The antidepressant drug Effexor XR™ and the anti-seizure drug gabapentin both do a nice job of reducing the frequency and severity of peri-menopausal and menopausal hot flashes and mood swings.

Vaginal lubricants such as KY Jelly™ may eliminate vaginal discomfort and dryness during sexual relations. Vaseline should be avoided if a condom is used as it reacts with latex and may result in leaks.

Vaginal estrogen may be used at bedtime once or twice a week to help with vaginal thinning and loss of lubrication. It is available in cream form or easy to use Vagifem™ tablets. Such treatment may also help with bladder control problems related to menopause. Vaginal estrogen used in this way is only minimally absorbed into the circulation and does not appear to be associated with increased risks.

All women, as they enter menopause, should have a bone mineral density (BMD) test to see if they have mild bone loss, osteopenia, or more advanced bone loss, osteoporosis. Although, at any given age, black women have higher BMDs than other groups, there are good reasons to believe that the bones of people with sickle cell disease are less dense and more fragile than those of others. These reasons include:

- expanded bone marrow cavities to replace red blood cells;
- delayed puberty, with fewer total years of producing adult quantities of sex hormones;

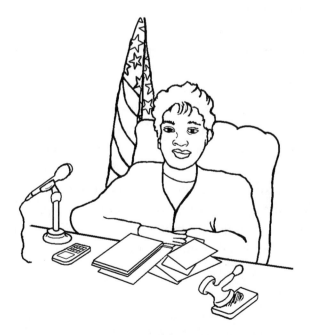

- less weight-bearing physical activity due to chronic and acute illness and lower average weight of people with sickle cell disease;
- more production of the stress hormone cortisol during bouts of acute illness;
- less production of sex hormones during acute illness; and
- bone loss due to bone infarction during pain crises and aseptic necrosis.

Today we have several non-hormonal options to treat and prevent bone loss and decrease the risk of fracture. Such interventions used in older women can be considered but have not been studied in sickle cell disease. These include the selective estrogen receptor modulator raloxifene (Evista™), the once-weekly bisphosphonates alendronate (Fosamax™) and risendronate (Actonel™), and the once-monthly bisphosphonates pamidronate and Boniva™. For folks who cannot tolerate these medicines or who have more severe bone loss, parathyroid hormone (Forteo™) may be used as a once-daily injection (like insulin).

Because vitamin D deficiency rates are higher among African Americans, levels should be measured or calcium–vitamin D supplementation should be considered. Of course, the foundation of osteoporosis prevention and treatment is calcium — 1,200 mg of elemental calcium/day for women before menopause in two or more divided doses with food and 400 IU of Vitamin D/day. After menopause, 1,500 mg of elemental calcium with food in three divided doses and 400–800 IU of Vitamin D/day should be taken.

An adequate diet should provide enough magnesium to help with calcium absorption, but if your diet is less than wonderful you should take a supplement of magnesium such as magnesium oxide. Vitamin K also assists with calcium absorption, but don't overdo it as it can also promote excessive blood clotting. Check with your doctor to determine what's right for you.

PREVENTIVE MEASURES

In this age group, the FARMS or preventive measures are the same as in chapter 12. Hydroxyurea can decrease the severity of sickle cell disease.

PSYCHOSOCIAL ISSUES AND SUPPORT

While adults will continue to benefit from peer support and support on the job, they will also be able, on the strength of their experiences, to help others in their practical and spiritual struggles. There is much you can do for yourself and for others:

- Develop hobbies and interests to distract yourself from daily pain.
- Get involved with fund-raising, or volunteering in the hospital that has served you.
- Become a mentor to a child or teen with sickle cell disease. Help others with school work.
- Be a camp counselor.
- Be a public speaker in your community.
- Get involved with politics to improve services for sickle cell patients.

This is a time to share your wisdom with the younger generation.

SPIRITUAL ISSUES

Patients with a solid spiritual foundation seem to do better physically and emotionally and are less depressive. Become involved in your local place of worship. People with a solid spiritual foundation experience less stress and fear of death. They also have a community of support when they are ill to help with family issues, transportation, meals, counseling, and encouragement.

PART THREE

LIVING WITH
SICKLE CELL DISEASE

CHAPTER FOURTEEN

Pain Assessment and Pain Management

INTRODUCTION

Of the many symptoms that can torment sickle cell patients, pain is one of the most common and distressing. This chapter tells you what you need to know about:

- the causes of pain;
- pain prevention;
- home treatment;
- emergency treatment; and
- in-patient treatment in the hospital.

We can't repeat it too often: *knowledge is power.* The more one knows about the causes, prevention, and treatment of pain, the better the chances of an early recovery. Certain types and causes of pain require a clinician's help and advice about treatment. Until recently, a doctor's assessment of a patient's pain could be quite subjective, and patients who were suffering were sometimes made to feel as if they were malingering, or even exaggerating pain in order to get drugs. Today, the Joint Commission on Accreditation of Healthcare Organizations (Joint Commission), the agency that inspects and certifies all U.S. hospitals, has issued new standards for pain assessment, treatment, and education. These new-pain management standards should improve the pain care sickle cell patients receive.

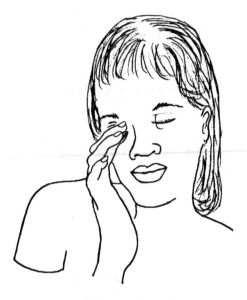

The most common acute problem of sickle cell disease causing presentation for acute treatment is the sickle pain episode (also unfortunately termed a pain "crisis"). A pain episode is defined as "a self-limited episode of diffuse, reversible pain often occurring in the extremities, back, chest, and abdomen." The severity of pain can range from mild attacks of five minutes to excruciating pain lasting days or weeks and requiring hospitalization. This intense pain is believed to be caused by the inflammatory response to bone or marrow death, or necrosis; reduced blood flow, or ischemia; ischemic muscle and ischemic bowel, resulting from the obstruction and sludging of blood flow produced by sickled red blood cells; or erythrocytes.

Although the pain episode is almost never a cause of death, affected individuals often fear serious complications or death. The frequency of pain episode varies with each person, depending upon his or her hemoglobin phenotype, physical condition, and many other variables. Trigger factors include events that cause increased physical and psychological stress, especially fever, dehydration, overexertion, rapid temperature change, or anger. Episodes, however, frequently occur without any apparent causes.

Recent studies in children and adults show that most acute pain episodes are successfully managed at home by individuals and their families. It is very important for the individual to learn how to manage his or her pain based on the type of pain the person is having and the severity of the pain. It is also essential that the individual know when he or she should immediately seek medical care for a pain episode. If he or she has fever, other illness, unusual or persistent pain, or vomiting that prevents the individual from staying hydrated, the individual should immediately seek medical care for the pain episode because other, more serious complications may be present.

The management of a pain episode begins with a complete clinical evaluation to exclude life-threatening complications, and to identify causes of pain that are not related to sickle cell disease. A detailed history and physical examination allows the doctor to identify treatable factors such as infection, dehydration, acidosis from any cause, emotional stress, extreme temperature exposure, or ingestion of other substances such as alcohol or other recreational drugs.

Because there are no characteristic findings that define the severity of a pain episode, *the patient's assessment must be accepted.* Treatment of a pain episode includes oral or intravenous hydration, analgesics, bed rest, and treatment of the underlying causes, such as infection.

RECORDING PAIN

It helps you and your healthcare providers to record the following information about your pain in a daily diary. Use the acronym **LOCATES** to locate the pain:

L—Location. Note the exact location of the pain, and describe if it "travels" anywhere.

O—Other Symptoms. Record any other symptoms like fever, nausea, or cough that come with the pain.

C—Character. Describe the pain. Is it deep? burning? throbbing? other?

A—Aggravating and Alleviating Things. What makes the pain better, and what makes the pain worse?

T—Timing. When did the pain start? Has it been there all the time, or does it come and go?

E—Environment and Effect. Where were you and what were you doing when the pain started? How does the pain affect your daily routine?

S—Severity. Be honest. If you always overstate your pain score, thinking healthcare providers will not treat you with enough pain medication, it could lead you to be over-medicated and have more side effects. Develop a sense of trust with your healthcare providers. They need to believe you and treat your stated level of pain with the appropriate amount of medication.

Pain scales should be available in the ER and the hospital. A scale you should be familiar with is the Visual Analog Scale or VAS. It is a 10-centimeter line with numbers from 0 to 10. Zero is "no pain," and 10 is "the worst pain you have ever had in your life." Mark on the line where you would rate your level of pain.

```
I_____ I_____ I_____ I_____ I_____ I
0        2        4        6        8        10
```

PAIN PREVENTION

For general pain prevention, remember FARMS. (Explained in detail in Chapter 2. Hydroxyurea can reduce the frequency of pain episodes.)

TYPES OF PAIN

There are five identifiable types of pain, each
with different treatments.

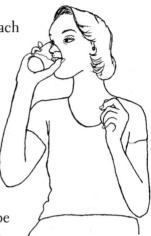

1. Acute sickle cell pain episode—pain
   that can last for several minutes to
   several days, caused by blocked blood
   flow from the sickled red blood cells.
   This pain is usually deep in the
   bones and muscles of the arms, legs,
   and back. Pain in the head, chest,
   or belly—or pain with fever—should be
   immediately evaluated by a healthcare
   provider.
2. Acute pain from another cause—pain that comes on suddenly and feels different from your usual pain episode should
   be checked by your healthcare provider. Pain in sickle cell
   patients may have other causes, such as stomach ulcers,
   appendicitis, a slipped disk, menstrual cramps,
   and so forth.
3. Chronic pain from sickle cell bone damage—pain that lasts
   longer than a few weeks and may be present daily. This
   occurs when bones are damaged by the blocked blood flow.
4. Chronic pain from other causes—daily pain that lasts more
   than six weeks caused by such things as a slipped disk, rheuma-
   toid arthritis, old injuries, and so forth.
5. Chronic nerve pain—pain caused by damage to the nerves
   from injury, sickle cell blockage, or other conditions like
   diabetes. Nerve damage causes a burning, tingling, numbing
   type of discomfort on a
   daily basis.

TREATING PAIN

1. Acute sickle cell pain episode. If this is a typical pain episode, note the type of pain and then start by drinking more water, lying down, and resting. Taking a warm bath can help, and so can distractions, such as music, TV, a game, or relaxation techniques. Massage to the area may be helpful. Or try moist heat (from a towel placed in warm water then wrung out).

If your healthcare provider has given you pain medication, start taking it as prescribed. Pain medications available without prescription include the following:

Acetaminophen (one trade name is Tylenol) will block fever, so do not use it until a healthcare provider has evaluated the fever and given the go ahead. Fever could mean a serious life-threatening infection is present. Acetaminophen is often combined with mild opiates like codeine (Tylenol 3™) or hydrocodone (Vicodin™). Be aware that these combinations will also block fever, and the amount taken must be limited to prevent taking too much acetaminophen that can damage the liver.

NSAIDs or *nonsteroidal anti-inflammatory drugs*, like naproxen (Naprosyn™, Aleve™) and ibuprofen (Motrin™, Advil™) block pain in the muscles and bones. It does not cause drowsiness. Again, it can block fever, so it must not be used until the fever is evaluated. Ibuprofen can cause stomach upset and ulcers. It is best taken after a meal or snack. It can interfere with the ability of platelets to stop bleeding from cuts. NSAIDs should not be used if there are kidney problems, stomach ulcers, bleeding problems, or asthma. This medication is good for menstrual cramps.

Aspirin has the same cautions as ibuprofen. One particular caution to note is that *aspirin has been associated with Reye's syndrome and should not be given to children with fever or cold symptoms.*

Codeine and *hydrocodone* are milder opiate medications that block pain in the brain. These medications are usually given in combination with acetaminophen or ibuprofen but can be given by themselves to block pain when a fever is being monitored. They will not block fever or platelets, and they don't cause stomach ulcers. These medications may cause drowsiness, nausea, and itching. They may also cause constipation, so be sure to drink plenty of water and eat plenty of fiber-rich foods like fruit, vegetables, and whole grains when using them. They are available by prescription only.

2. Acute pain from another cause. Pain in the head, chest, or abdomen and pain with fever should be evaluated; then the pain can be safely managed.

3. Chronic pain from sickle cell bone damage. The best treatment for this type of pain is not based on use of pain medications. The goal of treatment is not complete removal of the pain, because this is almost never possible all of the time. The goal of treatment is to reduce pain to a level that is tolerable and that improves quality of life and daily functioning. Strategies include change in behavior, physical therapy, weight loss, carrying less weight, transcutaneous nerve simulators (TNS), and mild heat. Long-acting arthritis medications are very helpful for daily pain control. The best medications for long pain relief, with the least side effects, are the arthritis medications called nonsteroidal anti-inflammatory drugs, or NSAIDs for short.

For long-term use, salsalate, celecoxib, and Mobic™ are safer for the stomach and duodenum than other arthritis medications because they are associated with fewer erosions and ulcers. There are now some serious concerns about several of the NSAIDs in that they may increase the risk of stroke and heart attack.

Opioid medications may be used with the NSAIDs if the pain is not controlled, or alone if the NSAIDs cannot be used. The long-acting opiates are morphine (MSContin™), oxycodone (Oxycontin™), or methadone. All of these agents block pain in the brain and cause drowsiness, constipation, tolerance problems, physical dependence, and physical withdrawal if they are suddenly stopped. Antidepressent medications used along with the pain medication help fight chronic pain. A stool softener to prevent

Pain Medications Available without Prescription

Name	Dosage by Weight	Notes
Acetaminophen Tylenol	20 lbs—100 mg 30 lbs—150 mg 40 lbs—200 mg 50 lbs—250 mg 60 lbs—300 mg 70 lbs—350 mg 80 lbs—400 mg 90 lbs—450 mg 100 lbs—500 mg 120+ —650 mg	• Use every 4 hours • Will block fever • Will not upset stomach • Does not block inflammation • Maximum adult dose 4,000 mg/24 hrs • Toxic doses damage the liver • May damage the kidneys and liver in chronic high doses
Ibuprofen Advil Motrin	20 lbs—100 mg 30 lbs—150 mg 40 lbs—200 mg 50 lbs—250 mg 60 lbs—300 mg 70 lbs—350 mg 80 lbs—400 mg 90 lbs—450 mg 100 lbs—500 mg 120+ —600 mg	• Give every 6 to 8 hours • Will block a fever • May cause stomach ulcers • May damage kidneys • May increase bleeding • Does block inflammation • Maximum adult dose 3,200 mg/24 hr • May increase blood pressure
Aspirin	Adults only 625 mg every 4–6 hours 80 mg per day to slow clotting down	• All of the same notes as ibuprofen • May cause Reye's syndrome in children— do not use in children.

constipation should be used when opiates are being taken daily. Tricyclic antidepressant medication, such as amitriptyline or certain serotonin reuptake inhibitors such as duloxetine (Cymbalta™) may work in combination with pain medication to help fight chronic pain. Muscle relaxants can help to reduce painful muscle spasm.

4. Chronic pain from other causes. All of the previous therapies listed are used to control chronic pain, as are nerve blocks and disease-specific medications.

5. Chronic nerve pain or neuropathic pain. Treatment with antiseizure medication has been helpful in pain control. Two such medications are gabapentin (Neurontin™) and carbemazepine (Tegretol™). Studies in patients with diabetic neuropathic pain suggest that tricyclic antidepressant medications, such as amitriptyline or certain serotonin reuptake inhibitors such as duloxetine (Cymbalta™), are also useful for this type of pain.

IN THE EMERGENCY ROOM (ER)

The emergency room (ER) is the next stop if home treatment fails or if there are danger signs such as:

- fever;
- weakness;
- atypical pain;
- headache;
- chest pain; and/or
- abdominal pain.

There are special emergency rooms for sickle cell patients in Atlanta, Ft. Lauderdale, Philadelphia, Baltimore, New York City, and other cities. At present, most sickle cell patients must seek out the emergency room with the best possible care. Some hospitals may not have staff members who are well trained in the care of sickle cell patients. The best defense is a good offense — come prepared with knowledge.

WHAT SHOULD HAPPEN?

Here, in a nutshell, is what you should expect when you go into an emergency room:

- First, your vital signs should be taken, including your temperature (normal 37.8ÞC or below); breathing rate (normal 15–20 per minute); heart rate—pulse (normal 60–100 per minute at rest); blood pressure (normal 90/60–120/80 at rest); pulse oximetry, a measure of the oxygen in your red blood cells (normal 95% to 100%); and your pain intensity score (how much pain you are having from, 0 to 10).

- A nurse should ask you about your main problem and assess how quickly you will be seen. In all emergency rooms, the most critical conditions must be seen first. A pain episode is not life-threatening, but there are symptoms that could require immediate treatment, such as fever, chills, headache, chest pain, abdominal pain, weakness, and abdominal swelling.

- A doctor, physician assistant, or nurse practitioner should examine you for signs of infection or complications. He or she should look in your ears, eyes, mouth, and nose, and listen to your heart, chest, and abdomen. He or she should also feel your abdomen for tenderness or swelling of the liver or spleen, and should check all of the areas that are hurting for swelling, heat, or tenderness.

- Blood tests, including a complete blood count (CBC), reticulocyte count, and chemistry values, may be done. A urine sample may be checked for blood, protein, and infection.

- Your doctor may have developed an individual treatment plan for you. Generally, an IV or intravenous line should be started with D5W sugar (dextrose) in water to rehydrate the sickled red blood cells. Generally, normal saline should not be used.

- Pain medication should be given through the IV if possible, and on a fixed time schedule based on the medication. Giving medication on a fixed schedule assures a good pain-fighting blood level can be reached and kept. If pain medication is given as needed or as requested, the pain relief is like a roller coaster going up and down. Pain medication given by patient-controlled analgesia (PCA) pump allows a continuous amount to go in all the time. You can use the pump button to give extra doses at a safe rate for extra pain control. Your pain should be reassessed periodically to see if the medication is working.

- Try to continue distraction therapy by reading a book, watching TV, listening to music, or playing a game. Relaxation techniques can be used.

COMMON MEDICATIONS USED IN EMERGENCY ROOMS

Many good pain medications are available for pain episodes, and many work better in combinations. Among those frequently used are the following:

- *Morphine.* Morphine is an opiate that blocks pain in the brain. It can be given by mouth, IV, in a patient-controlled analgesia pump (PCA), or by a shot in the muscle. Morphine takes effect in fifteen minutes and lasts up to three hours. It slows breathing down as the dose goes up. It can cause itching, nausea, vomiting, and constipation. The body can become physically dependent on morphine for several days after use. In coming off of morphine, the dose should be tapered off and not stopped suddenly.
- *Nalbuphine* (Nubain™). Nalbuphine is an injectable pain medication that is safe and effective in controlled doses. It does not slow respiration as morphine does. Nalbuphine has a "ceiling effect," so if it does not control pain as required, you must switch to another medication. This medication has fewer side effects, with less itching, nausea, and drowsiness than morphine. Nalbuphine may cause withdrawal symptoms in patients taking daily opiates (MS Contain™, Oxycontin™, Methadone™, and others), and it should not be used in those

patients. Nalbuphine is a great first choice for those not on chronic opiates.

- *Ketorolac* (Toradol™). This is an IV-administered, nonsteroidal anti-inflammatory drug that blocks pain in the bone and muscle tissue where the blocked blood flow from sickled red cells has caused damage. All of the cautions are the same as for ibuprofen. This medication can only be used for a maximum of five days continuously.
- *Meperidine* (Demerol™). This opiate pain medication is good for acute pain, but not for pain lasting more than a few days. It breaks down in the body to a substance that can cause seizures in high doses. This medication has all of the same cautions as morphine, which is a better first-choice opiate.
- *Hydroxyzine* (Vistaril™). In proper doses, hydroxyzine can prevent nausea and itching caused by opiates. It can also help calm fear.

PHYSICAL DEPENDENCY ON OPIATES

All opiate medications can cause the body to become dependent upon them after several days of continuous use. This is called physical dependence. The body then requires higher doses of the opiate to get adequate pain control. This is called tolerance.

If any of the opiate medications are used for several days and then withdrawn, the body will have withdrawal symptoms such as cramps, sweating, abdominal pain, and shakes.

Withdrawal can be avoided by slowly decreasing the amount of the medication used over several days to allow the body to adjust.

DRUG ADDICTION

Drug addiction is a complex behavior related to use of drugs on a regular basis to achieve effects not related to their primary effect of reducing pain. The diagnosis is difficult in someone with chronic pain or recurrent acute pain. True drug addiction can be diagnosed by the presence of a number of behavior characteristics including, but not limited to, devoting significant amounts of time and energy into compulsively seeking the medications; using the drugs for relief of anxiety or depression, or to get a high; and taking the medication when it is known to be harmful.

True drug addiction occurs in 5% to 10% of patients on daily opiates. At the Georgia Comprehensive Sickle Cell Center, we followed more than 2,400 sickle cell patients, and only 5% met the standard for drug addiction.

There is also a condition we call "pseudo-addiction." Patients who have been undertreated with opiates may experience uncontrolled pain and withdrawal symptoms. Some—indeed, too many—healthcare workers mislabel these patients as "addicts with drug-seeking behavior."

Until more sickle cell centers are available, patients with pain must keep returning to the ER for help. A good understanding of how opiates work and the proper doses of long-acting medications can stop this vicious cycle.

ADMISSION TO THE HOSPITAL

Admission to the hospital for more pain management or treatment is recommended within 48 hours of previous therapy, under the following conditions:

- if the pain does not decrease to a manageable level after 8–12 hours of treatment in the ER; and/or
- if a complication is present; that is, if you are experiencing a pain episode with any of the following:
  — infection;
  — temperature over 38° C;
  — pneumonia;
  — kidney infection;
  — blood infection (sepsis);

— low blood oxygen or too much acid in the blood;
— stroke;
— pregnancy;
— heart problems or failure;
— priapism that will not go away;
— blood clots in the lung;
— decrease in blood counts; or
— liver inflammation, gallstones, or gallbladder inflammation.

AS AN IN-PATIENT

After you are admitted into the hospital, treatment started in the ER should continue. There are several things you can do to ensure adequate pain management:

- Let the staff know your pain intensity level as a number from 0 to 10. Be honest and consistent, so the staff can provide appropriate treatment.
- Tell the nurses if you are having side effects like nausea, vomiting, constipation, itching, or feeling drowsy.
- Report your mood to the nursing staff. Feelings of depression, fear, anger, and sadness can all hinder your pain treatment. Counsel from chaplains, social workers, and nurses, as well as medication, can help in many cases.

Medication by patient-controlled analgesia (PCA) pump is one of the best options for pain control in the hospital. Report to your nurse any change in symptoms, or sites of pain.

RELAXATION TECHNIQUES

Pain can be helped by thinking about something else. Dwelling on the pain can make it feel worse. Being tense tightens muscles, reduces blood flow, and increases pain. Relaxation techniques help you relax muscles and get your mind off of the pain.

Start by getting in a quiet room, with some soothing music if it is available. Get in a comfortable position. Make a fist, release your fingers, and concentrate on letting them go limp. Tense your arm muscles, and then let them go limp. Tense your shoulders, then let them go limp. Tense your neck, then let it go limp. "Squench" your face muscles, and let them go limp. Tense your toes and feet, then let them go limp. Tense your leg muscles, and let them go limp. Tense your stomach, and let it go limp.

At this stage, all of your muscles should be more relaxed. If any feel tense, repeat, tightening and letting the tense muscles go until they are relaxed. Think of a calm place that you have visited, like a beach or park. Meditate on your favorite scriptures, song, or event.

Biofeedback, yoga, meditation, or hypnosis are other ways to help you to relax.

CONCLUSION

Discuss your pain-management plan with your healthcare provider when you are well and not in pain. Make a plan that is right for you. Keep this plan with you, after filling in the important information, to share with each healthcare provider you see.

There are free, problem-oriented guidelines for sickle syndromes available for healthcare providers on the Internet 24 hours a day at the Sickle Cell Information Center at *www. SCInfo.org*.

CHAPTER FIFTEEN

Managing Depression and Anxiety

People are at their best when each area of their lives is in a healthy balance. A steady decline in one's mood is evidence of depression. This can happen when facing the complications and pain of sickle cell disease. This low state of mood affects the body, the psychological and social state, and the spiritual outlook. Everyone, at some time in his or her life, experiences varying levels of negative feelings in mood due to internal and external issues or concerns; people can be sad and down for a brief time. However, disturbances in the mood that result in a clinical depression are so severe and ongoing that they require immediate attention and professional help, as well as positive support of available family and friends.

Fear or anxiety is a powerful emotion that causes the body to become charged to "run or fight." Constant fear can be harmful to the body, causing stress-related illnesses and even pain events. Naturally, people who live with daily pain often experience mood problems, such as anxiety and stress, insomnia, and depression. If chronic pain limits your ordinary activity, the problem can be even worse.

Some studies suggest that chronic pain causes the same changes in brain function as those brought on by stress. The body reacts to stress by putting out stress hormones, such as adrenaline. Such hormones allow our hearts to beat faster and our responses to be quicker when we need to cope with, or flee from, danger. In times of chronic stress, such as stress brought on by chronic pain, our bodies continue to put out more stress hormones than usual, even though there is no sudden danger from which we must run.

Constant increased amounts of stress hormones affect our bodies in a variety of ways. These hormones also can affect the mind. When you're stressed or in constant pain, your body doesn't produce enough serotonin, a chemical that helps to regulate several essential functions, such as sleep, mood, and anxiety. When you don't have enough serotonin, you are less able to fight depression, and, as some investigators believe, to deal with pain. That is why it's no surprise that people with chronic lower back pain are three to four times more likely to experience depression.

Depression can affect people with chronic pain in more than one way. Studies report the following:

- People in pain who are depressed are more likely to rate their pain as severe than people who aren't depressed.
- When depression is accompanied by sleeplessness, people experience more pain and other physical symptoms, as well as depression.
- People with chronic pain and depression more frequently have suicidal thoughts and attempts than people with other chronic medical problems.

Chronically depressed people often don't know that they're depressed. That's why it's so important to be evaluated by your physician, who can determine whether depression is complicating your chronic pain situation. Treating the depression may help improve some of the pain symptoms. (It is urgent that you seek help if you have thoughts of helplessness or of harming yourself or others.)

WHAT ARE THE SIGNS AND SYMPTOMS OF SEVERE DEPRESSION?

It is helpful to consider what happens to the whole person when attempting to identify troublesome areas of our lives. A holistic approach is exploring the components of the body, soul, and spirit. The body is composed of the physical areas of concern. The soul area is composed of the mind, will, emotional, and intellectual components that are involved in social relationships and environmental situations. The spirit is associated with the area of the inner being that is often connected with religious beliefs. Unhealthy balances are described in the following areas:

Body/physical disturbances in severe depression include:

- sleeping too much or too little;
- having trouble falling asleep;
- waking up early and not being able to go back to sleep;
- eating too much or too little;
- lacking pleasure in things you ordinarily like to do;
- lacking any fun in life; and
- withdrawing from normal life activities.

Soul/psychosocial disturbances that may be involved in severe depression are:

- life disruptions, such as job change, losses, family changes and relocation;
- problems with yourself, such as poor self-esteem, anger, shame, anxiety, increased self-destructive or suicidal thoughts, and an inability to concentrate; or
- problems with other people due to one's anger, irritability, arguments, social withdrawal, abuse, neglect, and/or excessive, extended grief.

Spiritual disturbances associated with depression can be:

- guilt and self-pity;
- fear;
- feelings of hopelessness;
- excessive worrying;
- isolation and loneliness;
- feelings of rejection, inferiority, and worthlessness; and
- feeling overburdened or unforgiving.

WHAT ARE SOME TREATMENTS TO CONQUER DEPRESSION?

The good news is that there are ways to return to a healthy balance in all areas in your life—and even achieve higher levels of improvements. The following are some suggestions that can help with depression of the body, soul, and spirit.

HEALTHY BODY BALANCE

Treatments for depression have also proved helpful when combined with chronic pain. Group programs, run by nurses with specialties in pain management, have been found successful. Such programs work without medicines, instead emphasizing education and behavior changes. Studies have shown that such programs reduce suffering and improve a sense of well-being even for people who have experienced pain for many years.

Besides joining a support group, you may also want to see a therapist (psychologist or psychiatrist). Chronic pain sufferers continually experience the losses that go along with daily pain, as well as the accompanying physical changes. A therapist can often be helpful by encouraging you to look at these losses closely, and to learn to cope with your feelings about them.

If your physician recommends an antidepressant, understand that he or she is not telling you that your pain is "all in your head."

The doctor is offering you an important tool for treating your pain. Many studies show that, even in people who aren't depressed, their chronic headaches, low-back pain, or diabetes-related neuropathic (nerve-ending injury) pain can be lessened through the use of antidepressants.

Commonly used antidepressants for pain treatment include older drugs, such as nortriptyline (Pamelor®) or amitriptyline (Elavil®). The best dose varies from person to person, and your physician will adjust your dosages to ensure that you are taking the amount that works best for you.

As to the power of the newer classes of antidepressants (SSRIs) to improve pain, the jury is still out. Some studies have shown improvement, while others have not. There is some evidence that venlafaxine (Effexor®) is at least as effective as the older nortriptyline class, with fewer side effects. Certain serotonin reuptake inhibitors such as duloxetine (Cymbalta™) have been shown to improve chronic pain caused by nerve damage in individuals with diabetic neuropathy. More work is needed to prove this in sickle cell, but, if one has chronic pain and is depressed, using one of these medications to treat the depression seems very reasonable. Other things you can do include the following:

- Have regular medical checkups, and immediate appointments when there is a radical change in physical functioning.
- Follow the medical plan and treatment of medical illness/disease, with laboratory and specialty consultations as needed.
- Get appropriate and supervised pain management by specialists with expertise in this arena.
- Have dietary and nutritional consultations and support to maintain optimal physical functioning.
- Report and discuss any new symptoms that may arise.
- Get your proper rest, relaxation, sleep, and exercise.

HEALTHY SOUL BALANCE

Balancing your soul involves three parts:

1. The "Phase of Life" Balance

- Attend to your needs and the needs of others as they come up so that they do not accumulate and become overwhelming.
- Obtain appropriate counseling support when you need help.
- Identify the sources of support for new circumstances.

2. The Relationship with Yourself

- Realistically identify your positive strengths and weaknesses, obtaining objective assistance if you are unable to do so independently.
- Spend quiet time with yourself so that negative feelings are not suppressed and ignored.
- Do something positive to deal with disturbing feelings and behaviors.
- Get immediate professional help and support from others who care about you whenever you begin to contemplate passive or active suicidal thoughts, plans, or intent.
- Seek help if you are advised to by caring family and friends— even if you can not see the need yet. Trust their judgment— especially when you know that you are not feeling right.
- Monitor your attitude, behavior, and habits, and keep them positive.
- Cease any behaviors that are abusive or neglectful of yourself or others. Do not be afraid to ask for help, or get help, when another advises you to do so.

3. Your Relationships with Others

- Avoid arguments, and strive for effective and positive communication.
- Settle disagreements quickly, and take accountability and responsibility for any problems you have caused.
- Maintain social contacts for support, recreation, and companionship
- Terminate any abusive or neglectful behaviors by another person. Do not be afraid to ask for help to do so.
- Talk to someone you trust when your grieving does not seem to get better or it seems to be getting worse. Get help if a loved one or colleague tells you that your grief is worsening.

HEALTHY SPIRIT BALANCE

Easing depression is the treatment for the body and soul. Your spirit needs tending to as well. Some suggestions to raise your spirits include the following:

- Monitor your attitudes and behavior, and do the "right" things—not violating spiritual guidelines, disciplines, or principles.
- Ask for spiritual support and guidance when you need it, such as times of struggle with helplessness, hopelessness, worry, fear, heaviness, or rejection.
- Accept spiritual support and fellowship from your community resources.
- Maintain a positive outlook. During times of distress and trouble, find hope through prayer, friendships, spiritual gathering, tapes, videos, etc.
- Focus on solutions, not problems.
- Practice being patient when going through difficult circumstances.
- Maintain the positives: in where you go, with whom you spend time, and what you spend your time doing.

- Seek out situations, environments, and people that increase your sense of security, safety, and support. Strive to be such a resource to others as well.
- Sing and listen to uplifting music.
- Practice fun hobbies and activities.
- Review and meditate on encouraging reading material, programs, plays, etc.
- Avoid talking negatively with others. Seek to maintain peacefulness.
- Avoid dwelling on thoughts and situations that bring fretting, fear, or anxiety.
- Maintain a thankful attitude for life.
- Avoid and/or terminate bad relationships, but cultivate those that promote love, compassion, understanding, accountability, responsibility, and growth.
- Seek wise spiritual counsel, helpers, and encouragers to get help during spiritual distress.
- Avoid situations that promote debt, fighting and arguments, divisions, and doubt.
- Set growth goals that get your thinking and behavior out of dysfunctional past behaviors, are progressively achievable, and that keep you being the best that you are meant to be.

Anxiety—which is bad enough all by itself—causes you to experience still more pain when mixed with chronic pain. The ability to feel "in control" of the situation can influence the degree of pain you experience. The more you know about what is causing your pain and how you can best control it, the less your anxiety and pain.

Because they know that anxiety makes pain worse, doctors often prescribe anti-anxiety medications for people with chronic pain. Medications used to control anxiety include tranquilizers in the benzodiazepine class, antidepressants, and antihistamine medications with anti-anxiety actions.

The benzodiazepines include diazepam (Valium®), alprazolam (Xanax®), and lorazepam (Ativan®), among others. They are effective in calming anxiety but, with regular use, can cause physical dependence. Antihistamines such as diphenhydramine (Benadryl®) or hydroxyzine (Vistaril®) have anti-anxiety effects without the posing dependence problems. Drowsiness is a possible side effect with either group. Buspirone (Buspar®), which is not a benzodiazepine, is specifically indicated for "generalized anxiety disorder."

As for nonmedication treatments, those proven effective include:

- counseling;
- distraction;
- relaxation exercises, like meditation; and
- music therapy.

CHAPTER SIXTEEN

Bone Marrow Transplant as a Cure

Keone Penn underwent the world's first unrelated cord blood transplant for sickle cell disease at Children's Healthcare of Atlanta at Egleston on December 11, 1998. Keone had been receiving monthly blood transfusions at Grady ever since he had a stroke at age 5. He had been coming regularly to the hospital ever since. Now, at the age of 24, Keone has become a pioneer.

Currently, the only curative treatment for sickle cell disease is a bone marrow transplant that completely replaces the patient's blood-making factory with donor cells. This is best done using a fully matched non-sickle brother or sister. Keone did not have a brother or sister match to donate non-sickle bone marrow, so the next logical step was to use an unrelated donor's blood stem cells from umbilical cord blood. Blood stem cells are very early cells that can produce every kind of blood cell when growing in the bone marrow.

Keone opened the door for the many sickle cell patients who do not have a sibling match but who have enough complications to merit the risk of the procedure. Twelve years after the transplant, Keone is free of sickle cell, but is still battling a number of complications, including the donor cells', attack on his tissues (a problem called graft-versus-host disease). Keone and his family are brave pioneers in the quest for a cure that may some day be available to all of those with sickle cell disease.

TRANSPLANTS: A PROBLEMATIC CURE

In addition to the treatments discussed, a cure for sickle cell anemia already actually exists. That cure is bone marrow transplantation (BMT). You might wonder why, if there is a cure, doctors still treat the disease with treatments that do not cure.

There are two answers to that. First, suitable bone marrow donors are not easy to come by. Second, bone marrow transplantation is itself a risky proposition. For sickle cell patients who have a matched sibling donor, the risk of death from the transplant procedure is about 5% to 10%, and there is also risk of serious infections, rejection, and graft-versus-host disease.

Furthermore, the donor runs risks with anesthesia and blood loss; these are much smaller, but still real, risks.

The high cost of bone marrow transplantation and follow-up care must also be considered. As you can see, this procedure is not a leisurely stroll through the park.

MATCHING TISSUE TYPES

Differing blood types (red blood cell incompatibility) is not a barrier to successful bone marrow transplantation, as it is for blood transfusion. But donor and recipient must be closely matched in tissue type, also referred to as HLA type. In general, the closer the two tissue types resemble each other, the better the chance of a successful transplantation. HLA testing is done on a blood sample drawn from the donor and recipient. An HLA-matched brother or

Bone Marrow Transplant as a Cure

sister, if available, is the best choice as a bone marrow donor. *In general, any two full siblings have about one chance in four of sharing the same HLA type.*

With respect to sickle cell anemia itself, the same genetic laws dictate that, if each parent carries one sickle trait, each child has a one out of four chance of having sickle cell disease (two traits), and a two out of four chance of having sickle trait. A sibling donor can have sickle trait but not sickle cell disease. Because of the difficulty of finding an HLA-compatible donor without sickle cell disease among one's own siblings, sometimes another family member, or an unrelated person who is HLA compatible, can donate bone marrow instead. This procedure would be more risky than using a matched sibling donor, and it is currently being studied in clinical research protocols at a number of transplant centers.

The National Marrow Donor Program (NMDP) has been developed to assist in the search for compatible unrelated donors in the United States. Unfortunately, there are relatively few African-American donors in the registry, making it difficult for African-American patients in need of a transplant to find a donor. For more information, contact the NMDP at 1-800-MARROW2 or *www. marrow.org*.

ELVIS'S STORY

Elvis Silva Magalhaes, at age 38, received a bone marrow transplant from his HLA-matched brother in Brasilia, Brazil. This made him one of the oldest people with sickle cell to have a BMT.

Elvis decided to have the bone marrow transplant after living for years with frequent pain and recurrent priapism. He also had leg ulcers. He recalls many sleepless nights because of sickle cell pain.

Today he is 42 years old and doing well four years after his bone marrow transplant. He says that he didn't know how good it could feel to live without sickle cell pain. His only medication is daily penicillin because of his functional asplenia. He is among the leaders of ABRADFAL, the Brazilian advocacy group for sickle cell disease. He stands up in international meetings to speak up for more services for sickle cell patients.

QUALIFYING FOR BONE MARROW TRANSPLANTATION

Bone marrow transplants are not undertaken lightly. In order to qualify for one, the patient, doctor, and family must do a great deal of preparation:

1. *Sickle cell eligibility*. Start by talking with your child's sickle hematologist. Whether the transplantation is appropriate to consider depends on whether your child has had severe enough sickle cell disease to justify the risks of bone marrow transplant. To help with the appraisal, the bone marrow transplant doctor will ask you about you child's medical history and look at the medical records, including the summary provided by your sickle hematologist. Important points to consider are whether there has been stroke and chronic transfusion, frequent hospital stays for pain or lung problems, or other major sickle cell problems. Once the medical information is received, a consultation with the BMT doctor can be scheduled.

2. *Other medical issues*. Make your doctor aware that your family is considering the bone marrow transplant option. The BMT doctor needs to know as much as possible about your child, including all medical problems, and whether or not they are related to sickle cell.

3. *HLA-typing blood tests*. HLA typing should be done on your child and the relative(s) with the highest probability of matching. Brothers or sisters from the same parents are the best potential donors, as long as they do not have sickle cell disease. HLA typing may be costly. Parents and half-siblings are unlikely to match unless there's an unusual family tree. If the sibling is not a full HLA match, then alternate donor transplant may be considered as part of a clinical research trial.

3. *Psychosocial assessment.* The patient and family's ability to cope with the challenges of a BMT is just as important as medical information and typing. BMT is a complex and demanding process, and a family unlikely to go through it successfully may be better off choosing other treatment options. Factors such as adherence (making appointments and taking medications), support systems, comprehension, and finances all play a role in the psychosocial assessment. A parent or adult family member must be available to stay with the patient in the hospital during the month-long in-patient portion. Once discharged, the patient must expect to stay near the hospital (within about a 30-minute drive) for several months, and come to the BMT clinic several times per week. The cost of BMT may be more than $400,000, and insurance may not cover all costs. The patient must be prepared to take as many as five to ten medications daily. All of these factors combined make transplant a challenging process. The BMT social worker, financial counselor, and other members of the patient and family support team will help with the assessment and with making plans for a successful transplant.

4. *Pre-BMT evaluation.* After all of the above steps are completed and decisions are made, scheduling the transplant can begin, which will be arranged by the BMT coordinator. A pre-BMT evaluation will be done over several visits. This includes medical testing of all the child's organs, blood tests and physical exams for both donor and recipient, and ongoing meetings with the BMT doctor to provide information and obtain informed consent. You should continue to ask all the questions you have. It is helpful to keep a notebook handy to jot down questions that come to mind.

THE TRANSPLANTATION PROCESS

Bone marrow transplantation can be described by dividing the process into three phases:

- preparation for transplantation (preparative regimen);

- transplantation; and
- post-transplantation management.

PREPARING FOR TRANSPLANTATION (PREPARATIVE REGIMEN)

A central venous line (a large IV) will be inserted in the chest; it can remain in place for weeks or months. This is so that the patient does not have to get pricked for IVs and blood draws. Before transplantation, chemotherapy and drugs that suppress the immune system are given to the recipient.

Chemotherapy drugs are commonly given to patients who have cancer. Even though sickle cell patients do not have cancer, chemotherapy is useful for the bone marrow transplant process by destroying the patient's immune system. This makes way for the donor's bone marrow to grow, and prevents the new donor marrow from being rejected. Chemotherapy drugs have many side effects. They are toxic to other organs in addition to the bone marrow. The BMT doctor will explain the side effects of the specific drugs chosen for your child's transplant.

TRANSPLANTATION

Donor bone marrow is usually taken from the large pelvic bones (back of the hips). The donor bone marrow is sucked out (doctors call this *aspiration*) with a special needle and syringe under general anesthesia, while the donor is asleep. The bone marrow is then given to the recipient intravenously through the central line. *The bone marrow stem cells* (the immature cells that will develop into the mature blood cell types) pass through the recipient's blood stream and find their way to the bone marrow cavities, where they will grow and mature if all goes well. Generally, two to four weeks are needed following transplantation before the transplanted marrow can produce enough mature red and white blood cells and platelets to sustain a healthy system.

POST-TRANSPLANTATION MANAGEMENT

During the weeks following transplantation, the patient needs to be isolated to protect against infection that can be life-threatening. Both bacterial and fungal infections can occur, but the infections can be treated with antibiotic and anti-fungal drugs. Painful mouth sores often develop, and intravenous narcotics are used to control pain. Platelet transfusions are necessary during this period to prevent serious bleeding. Packed red blood cells are transfused as needed until the new bone marrow can make enough red blood cells. If the donor and recipient are of different blood types, the blood type will change in the coming weeks.

NOURISHMENT

Chemotherapy often causes decreased appetite, nausea, and/or vomiting, which may make eating and drinking uncomfortable or even painful. These treatments may also interfere with stomach function and with the intestinal absorption of nutrients. Patients routinely require intravenous feeding. While intravenous feeding, or total parenteral nutrition (TPN), helps the host resist and overcome infections, it can also serve as an entryway for infections into the body. Scrupulous attention to caring for the intravenous feeding catheter and what enters it is, therefore, necessary.

SUCCESSFUL TRANSPLANTATION

The average time needed for successful bone marrow transplantation is six to twelve months, including preparation, the transplant, recovery, and intensive follow-up. Doctors determine the success of the transplant by blood and genetic tests. They will look at the hemoglobin electrophoresis to see how much sickle hemoglobin is left. A test called a chimerism will show how much of the blood is from the donor at any given time.

COMPLICATIONS

Complications may follow even otherwise successful bone marrow transplantation. Such complications include:

- graft failure (the new bone marrow does not "take");
- infection;
- graft-versus-host disease (GVHD), in which the donor cells attack the recipient's tissues;
- cardiomyopathy (a disorder of the heart muscle);
- veno-occlusive disease of the liver (blockage of liver veins causing swelling, fluid retention, and jaundice, which may be life-threatening);
- pneumonia or other lung disease;
- strokes, seizures, or bleeding in the brain;
- high blood pressure;
- kidney damage;
- infertility (inability to produce children);
- hormone dysfunction (early menopause, low testosterone, thyroid problems); and
- increased risk of developing cancer later in life. BMTs may also lead to cataracts (a clouding of the lens of the eye resulting in visual impairment). These are mostly the result of using steroids, such as prednisone, as part of the antirejection "cocktail." Steroids may also cause low potassium, bone loss, high blood sugar, mood and personality changes, kidney stones, and muscle wasting.

GRAFT FAILURE

Graft failure happens when the donor's cells do not successfully grow in the recipient's body. This may happen because of rejection (the recipient is fighting the donor), infection, not enough immune suppression, or problems with the donor cells (such as too few cells, or cells not closely matched enough). Sickle cell patients have a higher chance of graft failure than other BMT patients, such as those who have leukemia. Often the recipient's bone marrow will grow back, which means they will have sickle cell disease. It is possible that the bone marrow would not recover fast enough to fight life-threatening bleeding or infection, and death can occur. Graft failure may happen in up to 15% of matched sibling donor transplants for sickle cell disease.

ACUTE GRAFT-VERSUS-HOST DISEASE

Features of the Chronic Form of GVHD

- Skin rashes

- Inflammation of the corneas and conjunctivae (the outer lining of the corneas and the inner lining of the eyelids)

- Inflammation of the mucous membranes of the mouth

- Narrowing of the esophagus and inflammation of the intestines

- Respiratory (lung) failure

- Chronic liver damage

- Wasting (loss of muscle, fat, and bone tissue)

Acute graft-versus-host disease (GVHD) happens when transplanted white blood cells fight against the recipient's tissues (the host). Even when the donor and the host are completely matched, there are usually minor differences between their cells.

Acute GVHD usually involves the skin, the digestive system, and the liver. A skin rash is often the first sign. Diarrhea, abdominal pain, and intestinal paralysis may result from the intestinal involvement. Liver dysfunction may also occur. Severe immunologic deficiency may develop with a risk of life-threatening infection.

GVHD can usually be prevented or controlled with powerful immune-suppressing drugs, although these carry dangers of their own. It is essential that the recipient take the daily medication to prevent GVHD. Because GVHD can be debilitating and life-threatening, it is one of the main reasons that BMT is not offered to more sickle cell patients.; it is possible that GVHD may be as bad or even worse than having sickle cell disease itself.

THE FUTURE OF BONE MARROW TRANSPLANTATION

Research is now under way to expand the option of BMT to more patients, and to find ways of transplanting sickle cell patients without the high risk of complications. One approach is called *reduced intensity transplant*. This uses lower doses of chemotherapy in combination with powerful immune-suppressing drugs and sometimes low doses of radiation therapy. The main problem currently with this approach is the high rate of graft failure. If successful, this less toxic approach could make transplant safer and easier so that more patients could be cured.

Other efforts focus on using alternate donors in patients who do not have fully matched siblings available. The alternate-donor souce may be from cord blood, an incompletely matched relative, or an unrelated volunteer donor. The proportion of African-American donors must be increased to make this approach successful, and the NMDP has efforts under way to increase minority representation.

As reported in the Dec. 10, 2009, issue of the *New England Journal of Medicine*, a modified blood adult stem-cell "partial" transplant regimen cured sickle cell disease in nine of ten adults who had been severely affected by the disease. In contrast to the established method in children, this adult trial sought to reduce toxicity by only partially replacing the bone marrow. The much longer lifespan of normal red blood cells, compared to sickled red blood cells, allows the healthy cells to outlast and completely replace the disease-causing cells. Investigators used a low dose of radiation to the whole body and two drugs, alemtuzumab and sirolimus, to suppress the immune system. Alemtuzumab depletes immune cells, but does not adversely affect blood stem cells. Sirolimus does not block the activation of immune cells, but inhibits their growth, creating a balance that helps prevent rejection of the new stem cells. The radiation conditions the bone marrow, where donor stem cells move in and begin producing new, healthy red blood cells. After a median two and one half years of follow-up, all ten recipients were alive and sickle cell disease was eliminated in nine.

This new method of "partial" bone marrow transplant should allow many more sickle cell patients the opportunity to consider this as an option.

WHAT'S THE NEWS IN SICKLE CELL BONE MARROW TRANSPLANTATION?

Bone marrow transplantation offers a cure for sickle cell disease, but is only a good option for a small group of people. That group just got a little bigger when researchers at the National Institutes of Health announced early success with a new way to make bone marrow transplantation available for adults with sickle cell who were too sick for the standard ways of doing BMT.

Using the standard BMT approach was fatal for the majority of adults with sickle cell because their organs were damaged by years of living with sickle cell disease. BMT programs traditionally excluded adults, but the increasing life expectancy in sickle cell means there are probably more adults than children with sickle cell in the United States. Many doctors have been looking for new ways for adults with sickle cell disease to have safe and successful BMT.

The new approach from NIH features medications that heavily suppress the immune system—like kidney transplantation—instead of using the standard ways of doing BMT. Nine out of ten adults had successful transplants with this new approach, and they appear to be cured of sickle cell. The other one adult had graft rejection (the transplanted cells did not grow) and still has sickle cell disease, but the patient survived.

HOW GOOD IS THIS BREAKTHROUGH?

This is very good news, because it offers hope for adults to have cure by BMT, where standard BMTs were often fatal for adults with sickle cell. The 100% survival and 90% cure in these adults with the new immune-suppression approach are similar to the success rates in children with the standard BMT approach.

HOW COULD IT BE BETTER?

There is caution, because the long-term immune-suppression medicine may carry a higher risk of infections. Also, we need to watch for problems with graft rejection years later. Lastly, this new approach to BMT still requires a donor who is a full brother or sister and a very good match on tissue typing (HLA-match) plus either sickle trait or no sickle gene at all—the genetic probability of this combination happens in 18.8% of siblings.

HOW DOES BMT CURE SICKLE CELL DISEASE?

Because sickled red blood cells are made in the bone marrow, one way to cure sickle cell disease is to replace your own bone marrow with bone marrow from somebody else who does not have sickle cell disease. The major steps in transplanting bone marrow are:

1. finding the right donor (the best donor is a full brother or sister who is a complete match on tissue typing (HLA-match) and has either sickle trait or no sickle gene at all);
2. preparing the body to accept the new bone marrow cells;

3. releasing the new bone marrow cells into the bloodstream like a blood transfusion (not transplanted by surgeons)—these new cells find their way to the bone marrow space; and

4. waiting for the new cells to be accepted by the body's immune system, then grow and produce normal red blood cells instead of sickle cells.

In the standard preparation for BMT, medications wipe out the old bone marrow and make room for the transplanted new marrow cells to grow. Children can tolerate these medications and have successful cures by BMT about 90% of the time.

WHY CAN'T EVERYBODY HAVE A BMT? WHAT HAPPENS IF BMT IS UNSUCCESSFUL?

Steps 1 and 2 are huge barriers that prevent most people from having BMT.

1. The probability that your brother or sister has the right combination of genes to be a matched donor is only 18.8%, and not everybody has siblings at all. Doctors are exploring ways to use less-matched relatives as donors, or to find acceptable unrelated donors from the National Bone Marrow Registry or Cord Blood Banks.

2. The preparation to make your body ready to accept the transplant is very challenging, and doctors are still working to make the risks of BMT to be less than the risks of living with sickle cell disease. Currently, the standard BMT approach is offered for children who have had very severe sickle cell complications such as stroke or frequent acute chest syndrome or pain despite hydroxyurea treatment.

BMT can be unsuccessful in three ways:

1. graft rejection—you go through the BMT process, but in the end your own bone marrow grows back and you still have sickle cell disease;

2. graft-versus-host disease (GVHD)—the transplanted marrow attacks the rest of your body as foreign tissue and can cause great damage; or
3. death—can be caused by infection, bleeding, failure of bone marrow to re-grow, or damage to major organs (liver, lungs, kidneys).

CHAPTER SEVENTEEN

Hydroxurea Therapy and Hemoglobin F

Between conception and birth, our predominant hemoglobin is hemoglobin F (fetal hemoglobin). Having a high percentage of circulating hemoglobin as hemoglobin F protects against sickling and its many complications. We know this because infants with sickle cell disease do not usually have apparent problems until after about six months of age, when the levels of hemoglobin F have fallen substantially. Also, those with sickle cell diseases of Shi ancestry from Saudi Arabia, and patients from certain parts of India who have high levels of hemoglobin F, seem to get milder versions of the disease.

In short, a high percentage of hemoglobin F in a patient with sickle cell disease means that the patient is less likely to suffer complications.

The drug hydroxyurea has proven effective in raising the percentage of hemoglobin F by stimulating the production of protective fetal hemoglobin within the red cells.

Adult patients on hydroxyurea have 50% fewer pain episodes, 50% fewer blood transfusions, and 50% less need for hospitalization. Several studies in children have shown efficacy and short-term safety, and no bad effects on the child's growth and development.

The benefits of hydroxyurea are:

- decreased frequency and severity of pain crises;
- decreased frequency and severity of acute chest syndrome;
- decreased need for blood transfusions;
- longer life span ;
- less priapism; and
- possible weight gain.

For these and other reasons, an expert panel made a public statement in 2008 that hydroxyurea deserves to be more widely used for sickle cell treatment. (See http://consensus.nih.gov/2008/statement_sicklecell.htm.)

But there are also restrictions to its use. Because hydroxyurea, like other strong medications, has potential side effects, its use is reserved for sickle cell patients with the most problems. *Its safety for use in children with sickle cell anemia is now supported by many studies, but it is not officially approved by the FDA for use in children. Current studies are under way to show whether hydroxyurea use is safe and effective in babies and in milder forms of sickle cell disease.*

All available brands of hydroxyurea contain some lactose as a filler. About 70% of African Americans and a similar percentage of other groups prone to sickle cell anemia are lactose intolerant after childhood. Reactions may include:

- bloating;
- increased intestinal gas; and
- diarrhea and nausea.

Because hydroxyurea may harm or destroy an unborn baby, *a woman of child-bearing age must use a very reliable means of birth control while taking this drug.* If she is planning a pregnancy, she must stop taking this drug several months before attempting conception.

Because hydroxyurea is present in the breast milk of women taking the drug, *nursing women should avoid using it.*

Because hydroxyurea may also cause genetic changes in developing sperm cells and a decrease in the sperm count, *men should not take hydroxyurea for at least three months before attempting conception with their partners.*

Apart from the possible side effects already discussed, other rare but serious side effects of hydroxyurea, such as leukemia and skin cancer, can occur. Less severe, but more frequent, side effects reported in people taking hydroxyurea include:

- bleeding not due to low platelet counts;
- an increased frequency of infection;
- gastrointestinal disturbances;
- rashes;
- weight gain;
- hair loss; and
- darkening of toenails and fingernails.

Hydroxyurea should not be used if:

- your total white blood cell count is less than 2,500, because this could seriously reduce your ability to resist infection;
- your platelet count is below 100,000, because this could increase your risk of serious bleeding; or
- you have severe anemia, because your red blood cell count and hemoglobin could fall too low and your vital organs not receive enough oxygen.

LABORATORY TESTS YOU SHOULD HAVE BEFORE STARTING HYDROXYUREA

Before starting hydroxyurea, patients should have the following laboratory tests done:

- complete blood count, which includes hemoglobin, hematocrit, white blood cells, and platelets; and
- liver function and kidney function tests.

These tests need to be repeated frequently during therapy.

Patients taking hydroxyurea most often have to stop the drug to allow their low cell counts to come back up to a safe level (which usually occurs within two weeks of stopping).

MONITORING HYDROXYUREA

Complete blood counts must be done at least every two weeks while the patient is taking hydroxyurea. If the counts remain in an acceptable range, then the dose may be increased every 12 weeks over 24 consecutive weeks until the highest tolerated dose (35 mg/kg/day) is reached.

HYDROXYUREA FOR PATIENTS WITH IMPAIRED KIDNEY FUNCTION

Because hydroxyurea is mostly eliminated from the body by the kidneys, the dosage often has to be reduced in patients with impaired kidney function—unfortunately, a fairly common situation in patients with sickle cell disease.

ERYTHROPOIETIN IN COMBINATION WITH HYRDROXYUREA

The hormone erythropoietin (Aransep®, Epogen®, or Procrit®), which is normally made in the kidneys to increase red blood cell production in the bone marrow, may increase the effectiveness, and improve the benefits, of treatment with hydroxyurea. Hydroxyurea has helped many with sickle cell regain near-normal lives. Check with your healthcare provider to see if it might be an option for you. Like all medications, it may take a while to find the best dosage with the least side effects for your body. Know what to watch for so you can avoid complications.

CHAPTER EIGHTEEN

Gene Therapy for Sickle Cell Disease by Betty Pace, M.D.

E ffective treatment for sickle cell disease has developed slowly over the last 50 years, to the frustration of doctors and individuals living with the disease. But recent research progress shows how gene therapy holds promise as a cure in the future. Sickle cell disease is caused by a single change (mutation) in the building blocks, or bases, of deoxyribonucleic acid (DNA). The sickle mutation is in the beta hemoglobin gene found on chromosome 11. Hemoglobin is an important protein that carries oxygen from the lungs to other parts of the body.

In general terms, a cure for sickle cell disease can be achieved using bone marrow transplantation (see chapter 16) or gene therapy. Bone marrow transplant is already being used for a limited number of patients who have found a donor match. However, gene therapy offers hope for a universal cure that can be offered to everyone using a person's own cells. To understand gene therapy, a basic understanding of how DNA works is needed. Therefore the goal of gene therapy for sickle cell disease would be to repair the sickle beta gene or to add a normal gene in bone marrow stem cells.

GENE THERAPY TERMS

Bone marrow stem cells—Human bone marrow contains special cells, known as adult stem cells, that are needed to make all types of blood cells in the body (See Figure 1). Following a bone marrow transplant, these adult stem cells help correct the sickle mutation to bring about a cure. Bone marrow adult stem cells are different from embryonic stem cells that come from human embryos; the two cells should not be confused.

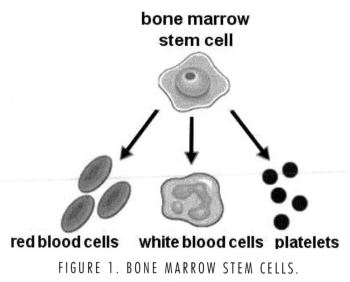

FIGURE 1. BONE MARROW STEM CELLS.

Stem cells are the source of all blood cell types in the body. They also can make a copy of themselves to keep a good supply of stem cells in the bone marrow. Hemoglobin protein is contained in red blood cells, and it carries oxygen to all other cells in the body. White blood cells help fight infection, and platelets are important to help stop bleeding from cuts or other injuries.

Genetic code—To understand gene therapy research, one must know about the genetic code. DNA contains the genetic instructions used to make proteins in living cells. Changes in the genetic code are also responsible for mutations that cause human disease. A mutation in DNA can lead to the production of a modified protein, such as hemoglobin S. One approach to gene therapy aims to correct DNA mutations, which in turn would correct the protein and bring about a cure.

WHAT IS GENE THERAPY?

Gene therapy is defined as the addition (insertion) or repair of genes in cells to treat genetic diseases, such as sickle cell disease. Human gene therapy is very complicated, and there is still much research that must be developed. Diseases caused by a single mutation like sickle cell have been the logical first choice for gene therapy treatment. However, problems involved in delivering large pieces of DNA to the correct place make this a slow process. Researchers are experimenting with ways to cure sickle cell disease by correcting the sickle beta gene or inserting a normal beta hemoglobin gene into bone marrow stem cells from sickle cell patients.

Types of gene therapy—There are two major types of gene therapy. Germ line gene therapy involves the correction or addition of normal genes to germ cells (sperm or eggs). The change would be passed on to later generations. This approach may cure genetic diseases, but it is not permitted in human beings for technical and moral reasons. The second type is somatic gene therapy, in which normal genes are added to somatic cells (cells in the body that are not germ cells). Any change in the DNA will only be to the person treated, and the change will not be inherited by later generations. This is the approach used to develop gene therapy for sickle cell disease.

Gene therapy methods—There are different ways to design gene therapy to treat human disease. The most common method is to add a new gene at a random location within DNA to make the normal protein. Other choices included swapping the mutant gene for a normal gene or repairing the gene mutation, both of which are very difficult to do.

HOW WILL GENE THERAPY BE DONE FOR SICKLE CELL DISEASE?

The most widely researched way to study gene therapy for sickle cell uses viruses. Through a natural process, a virus can stick to cells and place its genetic material inside the cells as a means of survival. From there they grow and cause disease. Taking advantage of this natural process, researchers have developed viruses that carry normal genes into human cells. To do this, the virus's genes that cause disease are removed, and then the human gene is added. This new combined DNA is called a viral vector because it will carry the normal gene into cells. The HIV virus has been used to make the most successful viral vectors for sickle cell gene therapy. However, unlike the HIV virus, the viral vector is not able to cause disease.

Research is also being done on other ways to produce a gene therapy cure for sickle cell disease. Non-viral vectors such as bacteria DNA, fat droplets, DNA by itself, or any combination of these have been used to add genes to cells. But their success has been limited. Our focus will be on the exciting progress made toward gene therapy using viral vectors.

GENE THERAPY OFFERS PROMISE OF CURE

Since the early 1980s, researchers have been working on gene therapy for sickle cell. Scientists have pursued two main approaches. Some are investigating whether correcting the sickle beta gene or adding a normal gene into adult stem cells will produce a cure. Another special approach involves turning off the sickle beta gene and turning on the fetal gamma gene (See Figure 2). Progress is being made, and there is a real possibility of a cure—but technical problems still have to be overcome.

The first major challenge was designing vectors that carry genes into stem cells and produce the normal hemoglobin protein. These vectors are now available.

A second problem was how to develop ways to isolate pure adult stem cells from the bone marrow, but this has been overcome. Once these two steps were achieved, then an animal was needed to test if the stem cells carrying the viral vector would cure sickle cell. Through the efforts of many researchers, in 1995 a mouse with sickle cell disease was made by two laboratories using the human sickle beta hemoglobin gene. This was a giant step forward in the field.

Chromosome 11

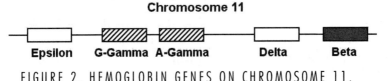

Epsilon   G-Gamma A-Gamma   Delta   Beta

FIGURE 2. HEMOGLOBIN GENES ON CHROMOSOME 11.

Five genes are located in the Beta locus. The two gamma globin genes make fetal hemoglobin during fetal growth in the uterus before birth. The beta gene takes over after birth to produce adult hemoglobin A. A person with sickle cell disease has a mutation in the beta gene and only makes sickle hemoglobin S.

The next major progress towards gene therapy for sickle cell happened in 2002, when researchers from Harvard University cured the sickle cell mouse using a lentivirus vector. Researchers removed bone marrow containing the sickle beta gene from the mouse and genetically "corrected" it by the addition of a normal beta gene (See Figure 1). The corrected stem cells were transplanted into other mice with sickle cell to produce a cure. Scientists are hopeful that the same treatment can be applied to human gene therapy using a procedure known as an autologous stem cell transplant, in which some of the patient's own stem cells would be removed, genetically corrected, and given back to produce a cure.

During that same period of time, French researchers tested the lentivirus vector on children with another disease called severe combined immune deficiency (SCID), also known as "bubble boy" disease. The children were cured of SCID, but a small number developed a leukemia-like condition. The study was stopped to:

- do more research to improve the vector;
- successfully treat the children for leukemia; and
- make new rules and regulations to ensure gene therapy for humans is as safe as possible.

Since that time, more children with SCID have been treated safely in many countries around the world with the new viral vector and cured. More important, they have not developed leukemia. The same viral vector will be used to treat sickle cell disease. The researchers at Harvard, working with the French group, have redesigned the viral vector with a modified normal human beta gene. They treated beta thalassemia first. If successful, then the same vector will be used to treat stem cell from patients with sickle cell. The research community is eagerly awaiting the results of these important studies.

Another group of scientists at St. Jude Children's Research Hospital, using the lentivirus vector, joined parts of the gamma and beta genes to cure sickle cell disease in mice. The gamma gene produces fetal hemoglobin, which blocks the problems caused by sickle beta hemoglobin. This design may work well in sickle cell patients. This study is in progress, but does not yet involve treating human patients.

There remains a challenge to collect enough stem cells from bone marrow or blood for gene therapy. In 2007, a group at the Whitehead Institute for Biomedical Research addressed this problem by developing a method to take skin cells (fibroblast) and treat them in the laboratory with growth factors to produce a new source of stem cells. These cells are called "induced pluripotent stem" or iPS cells. This new research was developed to cure sickle cell disease in mice, providing the first direct proof that skin cells can be used to treat a genetic disease. Much work is still needed before iPS cells can be used for human disease.

HOW WILL GENE THERAPY TREATMENT BE GIVEN?

The first application of gene therapy for sickle cell will be done with autologous stem cell transplant (See Figure 3). In this procedure, some of the patient's own bone marrow cells would be removed; the stem cells would be isolated and then genetically corrected. The patient's remaining marrow would be partially destroyed using drugs to "make room" for the genetically changed stem cells, which would be returned to the patient. Autologous transplant is less dangerous than the type of bone marrow transplant currently used to cure sickle cell disease, because the patient is receiving his or her own stem cells. This means the patient can avoid the complications produced by the body's immune system. More research is needed to determine the best way to achieve safe autologous stem cell transplant.

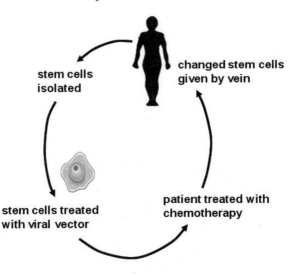

FIGURE 3. GENE THERAPY USING
AUTOLOGOUS STEM CELL TRANSPLANT.

The steps in this treatment include 1) isolating stem cells from bone marrow or the blood of sickle cell patients; 2) growing the stem cells in the laboratory; 3) repairing the sickle beta gene or adding a normal gene to the stem cells using a viral vector or other method; 4) testing stem cells to make sure the gene is working; 5) preparing the patient with chemotherapy drugs to kill the sickle stem cells in the bone marrow; and 6) giving the treated stem cells back to the patient to produce a cure.

Umbilical cord blood contains stem cells that can be used for gene therapy. The National Institutes of Health funded a study in 2001 to store umbilical cord blood from newborns with sickle cell with the hope that gene therapy will be available one day. The goal of this study is to develop the best way to store stem cells so they can be used many years later for treatment. This study is still open.

BARRIERS TO SUCCESSFUL GENE THERAPY

We still have a long way to go before successful gene therapy is achieved. Some of the problems to address are:

- the new gene does not continue to produce protein on a permanent basis — to be considered a true cure, there would no longer be a need to repeat the therapy;
- anytime a foreign material is put into human cells, the immune system will attack the invader
- viruses are the vectors of choice in most gene therapy studies, but they might produce side effects and interfere with other genes in the DNA;
- there is always the fear that, despite safeguards, the viral vector, once inside the patient, may recover its ability to cause disease; and
- if the vector enters the DNA in the wrong place it could cause cancer.

Ethical and legal issues are of great concern when discussing gene therapy. A review board known as the Recombinant Advisory Committee (RAC) was developed to address these concerns. Gene therapy could wipe out genetic diseases before they begin and eliminate human suffering; it has tremendous potential for the future.

However, there are many ethical concerns. First, it puts human fate in our own hands, giving scientists the ability to manufacture people. Some are concerned that gene therapy will be used to create a superior race. But the idea of gene therapy is to cure hereditary diseases, not to make any race superior. Another consideration is religion. Some consider it sinful to manipulate DNA. But somatic stem cell gene therapy is not passed to offspring; it allows the next generation to make its own decisions about medical treatment.

Some people feel that regulations will be hard to control, and gene therapy could become available on the black market. It could be used for any genetically linked trait such as your appearance or physical enhancement. Lastly, invasion of privacy is always a concern for many. Insurance companies could make it mandatory to have genetic screening before they issue a policy. This could cause discrimination against families with genetic diseases.

FUTURE OUTLOOK

Gene therapy has been progressing at a very slow pace, but this treatment is being tested for cancer, cystic fibrosis, diabetes, Parkinson's disease, and certain kinds of heart disease. Gene therapy has been ineffective and controversial, yet it is the most promising approach to curing genetic diseases. Like every other new medical advance, it will take time to develop.

Since the discovery of the DNA mutation in sickle cell anemia more than 30 years ago, the possibility of a cure has been the focus of extensive research. Until recently, advances in the development of gene therapy for sickle cell were held up by the lack of an animal model to test vectors, but this road block has been overcome. Ethical considerations continue to put a brake on research.

Several promising approaches to gene therapy have shown success in laboratory dishes of cells and in mouse models of sickle cell disease. Making the step to human gene therapy still has major challenges:

- delivering the gene to the right location;
- getting a large corrective effect from the therapeutic gene;
- avoiding side effects from the packaging system that delivers the gene therapy; and
- ensuring that the benefit lasts long enough to be worth the risks.

Gene therapy went to human trials in other diseases first (hemophilia, severe combined immunodeficiency, cystic fibrosis) where the technical challenges were smaller than in correcting hemoglobin genes. These clinical trials suffered setbacks, including deaths and leukemia, but brave patients continue to volunteer. As of this writing, the first gene therapy trial for sickle cell disease and thalassemia has enrolled two patients with hemoglobin E beta-thalassemia in Paris, France. Gene therapy was rejected in the first patient, but the second has become transfusion-free and is doing well 27 months after the gene therapy.

Although much work remains, the future promises better and safer gene therapy tools and even an eventual cure.

CHAPTER NINETEEN

Participating in Sickle Cell Research

E ven as you read this, people across the world are working to find new medications and treatments for sickle cell disease. This research goes on in the form of "clinical trials," in which new medications and methods are tested both for their effectiveness and their safety. Sickle cell patients and families should consider helping find new treatments that will improve many lives, including there own. Without patients willing to participate, there will be no new advances in sickle cell treatment.

Patients who take part in such studies do better than patients who do not, because the study provides expert medical care, the latest information, free lab studies, and free treatment. To find the latest research in a particular area, go to the Web site *www. ClinicalTrials.gov*. Do a search on the words *"sickle cell"*. You may also contact your nearest medical school or university, or your primary care provider, to learn about research going on in your area.

PLACEBO EFFECT

Some trials will be designed to explore the power of the mind to strengthen and heal the body. In such trials, some patients will be given the active medication being explored, but others will be given a placebo. A placebo is an inactive pill, liquid, or powder

Clinical Trials: Benefits and Risks

The benefits of participating in clinical trials are that you:
- play an active role in your health care;
- gain access to new research treatments before they are widely available;
- obtain expert medical care at leading healthcare facilities during the trial; and
- help others by contributing to medical research.

The risks involved in clinical trials include:
- possible unpleasant, serious, or even life-threatening side effects to treatment; and
- the chance that a treatment may not work for you.

that looks like the real medication, but has no treatment value. The other way to see if new treatments are effective is to have a "control" group that gets the standard treatment.

AN INTRODUCTION TO CLINICAL TRIALS

Choosing to participate in a clinical trial is an important personal decision that most people don't want to make alone. Instead, they talk to their physician and to family members or friends before deciding. Once you have identified trials that might help you, contact the study research staff and ask questions about these trials. That way, you'll know that the decision you make will be a good one. Next, you would like to review the protocol for the clinical trial.

WHAT IS A PROTOCOL?

A protocol is a study plan on which all clinical trials are based. The plan is carefully designed to safeguard the health of the participants as well as to answer specific research questions. A protocol describes what types of people may participate in the trial; the schedule of tests, procedures, medications, and dosages; and the length of the study. While they are in a clinical trial, participants following a protocol are seen regularly by the research staff for the purpose of monitoring their health and determining the safety and effectiveness of their treatment.

WHAT ARE THE DIFFERENT TYPES OF CLINICAL TRIALS?

Treatment trials test new treatments, new combinations of drugs, or new approaches to surgery or radiation therapy.

Prevention trials look for better ways to prevent disease in people, or for ways to prevent a disease from returning. These approaches may include medicines, vitamins, vaccines, minerals, or lifestyle changes.

Screening trials test the best way to detect particular diseases or health conditions.

Quality of life trials (or supportive care trials) explore ways to improve the comfort and quality of life of people who must live with a chronic illness.

WHAT ARE THE PHASES OF CLINICAL TRIALS?

Clinical trials are conducted in phases. The trials at each phase have a different purpose and help scientists answer different questions:

- In *Phase I trials*, researchers test, for the first time, a new drug or treatment in a small group of people (20 to 80) to evaluate its safety, determine a safe dosage range, and identify side effects.
- In *Phase II trials*, the drug or treatment is given to a larger group of people (dozens or hundreds) in order to find out more about its safety and effectiveness.

- In *Phase III trials*, the study drug or treatment is given to large groups of people (hundreds or thousands) to confirm its effectiveness, monitor side effects, compare it to commonly used treatments, and collect information that will allow the drug or treatment to be used safely.
- In *Phase IV trials*, drugs or treatments already approved by the Food and Drug Administration are studied to find additional information, including risks, benefits, and optimal use.

WHAT HAPPENS DURING A CLINICAL TRIAL?

The trial team includes doctors and nurses as well as social workers and other health care professionals. They check the health of the participant at the beginning of the trial, give specific instructions for participating in the trial, monitor the participant carefully during the trial, and stay in touch after the trial is completed.

Some clinical trials involve more tests and doctor visits than the participant would normally have for an illness or condition. For all types of trials, the participant works with a research team. Frequent contact with research staff members yields the best likelihood of a good outcome.

WHAT IS INFORMED CONSENT?

Informed consent means that, before you decide whether or not to participate in a clinical trial, you've learned the key facts about it. It is also means that you will be given further information during each stage of the trial.

To help you decide whether or not to participate, the doctors and nurses involved in the trial explain it in detail. If your native language isn't English, a translator can be provided. It is the researcher's responsibility to explain it in a way that you understand.

Once you have understood the explanation, you'll be given an informed consent document that includes details about the study, such as, its purpose, duration, required procedures, and key contacts. Risks and potential benefits are also explained in the document. Then the researcher of staff member will ask if, you're ready to decide whether or not to sign the document. Informed consent is not a contract, and the participant may withdraw from the trial at any time.

WHAT ARE SOME KEY ISSUES YOU SHOULD DISCUSS WITH THE TRIAL TEAM?

The team will want you to know as much as possible about the clinical trial and feel comfortable asking questions. You'll want to know what care you'll be provided while the trial goes on, and what part, if any, of the trial treatment you will have to pay for.

The following are the kinds of questions you'll want answers to. (Some of the answers to these questions are found in the informed consent document.)

- What is the purpose of the study?
- Who is going to be in the study?
- Why do researchers believe the new treatment being tested may be effective? Has it been tested before?
- What kinds of tests and treatments are involved?
- How do the possible risks, side effects, and benefits in the study compare with those of my current treatment?
- How might this trial affect my daily life?
- How long will the trial last?
- Will hospitalization be required?
- Who will pay for the treatment?
- Will I be reimbursed for other expenses?
- What type of long-term follow-up care is part of this study?
- How will I know that the treatment is working?
- Will results of the trials be provided to me?
- Who will be in charge of my care?

The protocol may require more of your time and attention than you can give.

HOW SAFE IS THE TRIAL?

The ethical and legal codes that govern medical practice in general also apply to clinical trials. Most clinical research is federally regulated and monitored, with built-in safeguards to protect you throughout the course of the trial. The trial follows a carefully controlled protocol—a study plan that lays out in detail what the researchers will do in the study.

Your protection doesn't stop there. While the trial is going on, your team will report results at scientific meetings, publish interim findings in medical journals, and also report interim findings to various government agencies.

In addition, every clinical trial in the United States must be approved and monitored by an institutional review board (IRB) to make sure the risks are as low as possible, as measured against the disease itself. An IRB is an independent committee of physicians, statisticians, community advocates, and others who work to ensure that a clinical trial is ethical and that the rights of study participants are protected. By federal regulation, all institutions that conduct or support biomedical research involving humans must have an IRB that initially approves and periodically reviews the research.

In a Nutshell

People, and especially minorities, sometimes avoid clinical trials because they fear they will be "experimented on." In fact, doctors and clinics that conduct clinical trials are usually the best in their field, and can offer you the best possible care with the latest treatment. Participating in a trial will lower your costs and provide you with services you might otherwise not have been able to get. Check out the facts about clinical trials that could help you make an informed decision.

CHAPTER TWENTY

What You Can Do

THE POWER OF ONE

Twenty-five years ago in Atlanta, when her son Carey was eight, doctors told Berrutha Harper that her son would die before his teen years of sickle cell disease. Berrutha had to take her son to the local emergency rooms for pain treatment, and she often experienced long waits and had to deal with health care providers who had little or no sickle cell experience.

When Berrutha saw that she couldn't get consistently good care in ordinary emergency rooms, she began to dream of an emergency room dedicated to the needs of sickle cell patients, with a specially trained staff of healthcare providers who would treat patients with knowledge and compassion.

Berrutha was the kind of dreamer who saw a dream as possibility. She organized other parents and patients into a group of people who could share concerns about sickle cell patients and consider how to improve sickle cell care in the largest of the Atlanta hospitals, Grady Memorial.

The hospital received many patient complaints each day about the care given to emergency room sickle cell patients. But the hospital's official position was that it couldn't afford an emergency room dedicated exclusively to the treatment of sickle cell patients.

Berrutha was not the kind of woman to give up easily. She set out to get state funding from the legislature. During lunch breaks from her job as a medical clerk in a local healthcare clinic, she would go to the state capitol building and knock on legislators' doors.

One day, a patient came into the emergency room with chest pain, and was treated for sickle cell pain crisis. The patient died of a heart attack, a diagnosis not thought of because the patient had sickle cell disease. Berrutha called all of the parent/patient groups to stage a protest march in front of the state capitol. Berrutha arrived at the capitol with signs in hand, but no people showed up to march. A discouraged Berrutha sat on the steps and sent up a short prayer. A group of school bus drivers from south Georgia, who had delivered school children for a capitol tour, asked Berrutha about the protest signs and got an education about sickle cell disease. The bus drivers asked if they could carry the signs for Berrutha, as they would be there waiting for the school kids to return. The news of the marching bus drivers reached the inner chambers of the legislators in session. The leader of the Black Caucus came outside and invited Berrutha to meet with him if she would call off the march. This was the first time Berrutha's story was heard by the influential leaders of the legislature. Funds were allocated to Grady Memorial Hospital to start a 24-hour clinic with a dedicated staff of healthcare providers trained to care for sickle cell patients.

In September 1984, the Sickle Cell Center opened its doors for patients. It has been open ever since, providing round-the-clock emergency care, comprehensive preventive care, research, in-patient consultations, and education. All of this was the result of one mother's prayer, vision, and perseverance.

FUND-RAISING

There are several ways to raise money for your sickle cell activities. First, set up or partner with a 501(c)(3) tax-exempt organization so donations can be tax-deductible. Many hospitals, churches, and civic groups have this status. Plan a budget. Funds will be needed for scholarships for college, emergency needs of patients, research projects, and education. Fund-raising activities include 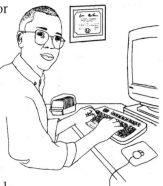 walk-a-thons, bowl-a-thons, banquets, and concerts. Invite corporate participation, and invite the local press to do a story on the event. This will raise awareness about sickle cell disease and raise funds at the same time.

BLOOD DRIVES

It is important to reduce the formation of antibodies in sickle cell patients. The best way to do this is to transfuse blood from people of the same ethnic background. If sickle cell disease primarily effects those in the African-American community in your area, then blood donations should be increased in that community to reduce the antigen exposure. The more antibodies a patient makes, the more difficult it is to find blood that matches and will not cause a transfusion reaction.

Get involved by organizing a blood drive in your civic or church group. Contact the local Red Cross chapter, which can help you set up a blood drive. Ask about a Partner for Life program, in which a group of donors can be matched to a specific sickle cell patient to reduce the blood exposure and reduce the making of antibodies. At the blood drives, educate the public about sickle cell disease and the need for regular blood donations.

BONE MARROW REGISTRY

The National Marrow Donor Program at *www.marrow.org* helps organize testing for potential bone marrow donors. As transplants increase as options for sickle cell patients, a larger list of potential donors will increase the success of finding a match. This program is great to offer while doing blood drives and helps raise awareness of sickle cell disease.

HEALTH FAIRS

Health fairs are good places to educate the public about sickle cell disease. Set up a table with informational handouts, and have people on hand to answer questions. If possible, provide sickle cell screenings by drawing blood for hemoglobin electrophoresis. You can network with other community-based health organizations to help support sickle cell patients.

PUBLIC EDUCATION

Educate the public in your community by inviting the local newspaper and TV news to do stories about patients and events in your area. Sickle cell patients have wonderfully inspirational life stories of overcoming pain and hardship. Talk about innovative support groups or new advances in research.

POLITICS

Tell your legislators about sickle cell disease and the need for services in your community. States can be involved in newborn screening, funding comprehensive centers, funding vocational-rehabilitation programs, and funding preventive care. You can contact legislators by newsletters, personal calls, personal visits, and e-mail. Invite them to your educational events. National leaders need to be educated about the unique needs of sickle cell patients and the need for increased research funding. Sickle cell is the second most common genetic disease in the United States, but it is underfunded compared to other, less common genetic diseases such as hemophilia and cystic fibrosis.

Make the Most of Your Meeting with Legislators or Their Staff

You have an appointment with a legislator, executive, or legislative aide—Congratulations! You will probably have a limited time, only 15 to 30 minutes, so you want to be prepared to make the most of this time! Here are suggestions to help you have a successful meeting.

Coordinate your advocacy efforts with others—it will be a stronger message for action if many groups of people unify to advocate the same goals for sickle cell rather than if each person suggests a different goal.

Thank them for their support for Americans suffering from sickle cell disease. This is a good way to start off the meeting positively and will show them that you appreciate their efforts.

Prepare an outline of your message: the "talking points." If you are coming as a group, assign each person to speak about one point.

o Tell your story. Prepare personal stories and anecdotes to share.

o Make the case for one or two goals. Give statistics from your community that illustrate why the current funding does not meet the need.

o Ask for a commitment to support increased funding for sickle cell. Your goals are to enlist support for the next fiscal year's funding requests as well as the long-term support of sickle cell treatment and research programs. It is important to be as specific as you can.

Thank them for the meeting, and follow-up promptly. Let them know that you appreciate their work and taking the time to meet with you. Send them any information or materials that you promised during the meeting.

If you meet with an aide or other staff member, be respectful and do not be discouraged. Legislators depend on their staffs to help them keep track of the numerous issues that are important to the communities they represent. Legislative aides are often very knowledgeable on your issues, and they have substantial influence over their legislator. Regardless of their title or age, they can help make policy decisions and can be very important allies in helping victims.

The same approach can be used for letters or other communication, even if it is not a face-to-face meeting.

Adapted from a Sickle Cell Disease Association of America handout.

SICKLE CELL CAMP

Many sickle cell centers and foundations in major cities have annual sickle cell summer camps for children. Camp is a way for children to interact with their peers in a fun environment. Usually, medical support is provided by the medical teams from the sickle cell centers. Campers are encouraged to drink extra fluids, take rest breaks, and avoid high-temperature exposure. These camps typically charge a small fee to cover lodging and food. Frequently, scholarships are provided to those who do not have any resources. To locate a camp, contact the nearest sickle cell center or the Sickle Cell Disease Association of America for the chapter nearest to you.

WHY SUPPORT AND COUNSELING ARE VITAL

Sickle cell disease is not only an anemia of the blood. Like all serious illnesses it affects every aspect of the patient's life, and the physical ills can be made worse by intense emotional and social stress. Without proper medical attention and support from those organized to help, the psychological component of this disease can prove to be as devastating as the disease itself.

In some respects, better treatment and care of sickle cell patients have intensified the emotional and psychological problems associated with the disease. Because life expectancies have increased, patients can face a seemingly unending prospect of absence from school and work, poor employment prospects, and managed-care crises. Depression, boredom, and antisocial or self-destructive behaviors are expressions of the intense emotional strain the patient faces daily.

The very good news is that sickle cell patients don't have to face the disease alone. From initial screening through every stage and pain episode, counseling and support are available. One only has to look.

Not only is immediate help available to the patient, but counseling and support are also there for family, friends, teachers, employers, and healthcare professionals. In fact, the interconnected efforts of the entire sickle cell community are key to successful support.

What we offer you here, to start you on your journey, is a basic list of the resources that will get you started. Once you take the first step, you'll find that the appropriate path will be obvious. Simply walk it, as you do any walk, one step at a time.

What you will soon see is that each organization is a link in a long, interconnected chain of support, a chain that has grown much stronger in the past 30 years, as we have all come to better understand the needs of the sickle cell patient.

Once you start, you'll soon find that there are different kinds of support groups available:

- Some agencies are government-sponsored, but many are community-based.
- Some focus on education and clinical research for the medical community.
- Some stress political activism in their efforts to generate the funds for clinical research and community-outreach programs.
- Others stress one-on-one personal involvement and individual care.

Whatever the approach, their goal is the same—to fight for the health and rights of the individual sickle cell patient.

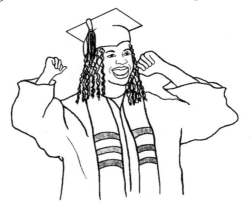

CHAPTER TWENTY-ONE

Resources

NATIONAL ORGANIZATIONS

In 1972, in a key step toward greater sickle cell disease awareness, the National Institutes of Health (NIH) created Comprehensive Sickle Cell Centers (CSCCs). Although their main emphasis is clinical research, the CSCCs provide the community services such as screening, counseling, and education.

Ten CSCCs were funded at a time, and the list of centers would change every 5 years because of the federal government's funding cycles. The NIH stopped funding the CSCCs in April 2008. About 30 medical centers still follow the comprehensive sickle cell centers model. Clinical research continues, and is organized in several overlapping networks of these sickle cell centers. However, the support for the community services like screening, counseling, and education is uncertain. A list of clinics is maintained at *www.SCInfo.org/clinics.htm.*

KEY COMMUNITY ORGANIZATIONS ON THE WEB

The World Wide Web is an invaluable resource for researching sickle cell support groups. Key organizations, such as the American Sickle Cell Anemia Association (ASCAA), the Sickle Cell Disease Association of America (SCDAA), and the Sickle Cell Information

Center, have links nationwide. The Sickle Cell Society is based in London, England, to help patients and families in Europe. These groups are working to raise awareness of the needs of the sickle cell patient while reaching out to patients and families.

MEDICAL INFORMATION ON THE INTERNET

There are hundreds of Web sites offering medical information on the Internet. Many sites offer wonderful information, while other sites do not. You need to judge the credibility of the information on the Internet by using a few simple rules:

1. Who is the author of the information? You can look at the last three letters of the Web site and see .gov for U.S. government sites like NIH.gov and CDC.gov. Those ending in .edu are sponsored by educational institutes like universities. Those ending in .org are usually non-profit organizations.
2. Is there an editorial board that oversees the information? This should include physicians and other healthcare providers.
3. Is the site selling you a medication or treatment? Are there excessive commercials within the site? Be wary of bias in the information.
4. Is the information current? Check the dates of the information.
5. Is your privacy being protected? Be wary of sites that want too much personal information before they give you information.

See if the Web site is a member of Health on the Net (HON): *www.hon.ch/HONcode.*

The American Sickle Cell Anemia Association

This organization provides a wide range of services to people with either sickle cell trait or variants of the disease itself—and to their families. Key services include ongoing follow-up diagnostic testing, counseling, and tracking services for parents with infants who screen positive; family counseling and support services; coordination of medical and social services, education, and support for the program's clientele; teacher education; and screening services at upwards of 75 local health fairs. In addition, ASCAA has outreach programs to the region's African-American, Hispanic, Mediterranean, and Arab communities for family education and the identification of incidence of sickle cell disease.

American Sickle Cell Anemia Association
P O. Box 1971
10300 Carnegie Avenue
Cleveland, OH 44106
216-229-8600
216-229-4500 fax
www.ascaa.org

The Sickle Cell Disease Association of America

The goal of the Sickle Cell Disease Association of America (SCDAA) is "to find a cure and improve the quality of life for those who are afflicted and their families." The SCDAA publishes and distributes to parents and teachers educational materials for living and coping with sickle cell disease.

Through its member organizations, SCDAA provides such services as screening and referrals, counseling, home nursing care, research updates, psychosocial services, transportation, summer camp, local and regional workshops, international symposia, as well as a sickle cell chat room. The SCDAA also provides guidelines for starting local sickle cell groups.

Sickle Cell Disease Association of America
231 East Baltimore Street
Suite 800
Baltimore, MD 21202
800-421-8453
410-528-1555
410-528-1495 fax
www.sicklecelldisease.org
E-mail: scdaa@sicklecelldisease.org

The American Society of Hematology

This is the national organization supporting hematologists (blood experts). They support sickle cell research, publications, and professional education. They have an annual meeting at which many sickle cell research results are presented.

American Society of Hematology
2021 L Street NW
Suite 900
Washington, DC 20036
202-776-0544
202-776-0545 fax
www.hematology.org

The Sickle Cell Society of London, England

This is an international sickle cell organization based in England that supports patient and professional education.

Sickle Cell Society
54 Station Road
London
NW10 4UA
UK
020-8961-7795
020-8961-8346 fax
www.sicklecellsociety.org

International Association of Sickle Cell Nurses and Physician Assistants (IASCNAPA)

IASCNAPA is an association of nurses, physician assistants, and other healthcare workers caring for sickle cell patients worldwide. www.iascnapa.org

The Alliance of Genetic Support Groups

This nonprofit health-advocacy organization is committed to transforming health through genetics.

The Alliance of Genetic Support Groups
4301 Connecticut Avenue NW
Suite 404
Washington, DC 20008
800-336-4363
202-966-5557
202-966-8553 fax
www.geneticalliance.org
E-mail: info@geneticalliance.org

National Heart, Lung, and Blood Institute (NHLB)

The NHLB is a part of the federal government's National Institutes of Health, focused on research, training, and education programs to promote the prevention and treatment of heart, lung, and blood diseases.

Sickle Cell Disease Scientific Research Group
6701 Rockledge Drive, MSC 7950
Bethesda, MD 20892
301-435-0055
301-480-0868 fax
www.nhlbi.nih.gov

St. Jude Children's Research Hospital—Sickle Cell program

St. Jude's provides comprehensive treatment, conducts research, and provides clinical trials in its sickle cell program.

St. Jude Children's Research Hospital
262 Danny Thomas Place
Memphis, TN 38105
901-595-3300
www.stjude.org/phecom

Sickle Cell Information Center

This is a comprehensive sickle cell site based at the Georgia Comprehensive Sickle Cell Center at Grady Health System in Atlanta, Georgia. In 1984, Grady Memorial Hospital opened the world's first 24-hour comprehensive acute care Sickle Cell Center. The goals of the center were to provide 24-hour acute care in a designated area with a dedicated staff, provide healthcare consultations, research new treatments, and provide education and support services to residents of the state of Georgia with sickle cell syndromes. The mission of the Web site is to provide sickle cell patient and professional education, news, research updates, and worldwide sickle cell resources. E-mail consultations are now provided to patients and clinicians in countries around the world. All e-mail questions are reviewed by a physician assistant and answered or sent to the appropriate medical staff member for a reply.

Current content areas include: sickle cell overview for the lay audience, an overview for providers, research updates, a list of sickle cell clinics and centers, Web links, a downloadable PowerPoint tutorial, a frequently asked questions page, and a means of submitting e-mail questions. The Web site contains sections for healthcare providers, including two online clinical-management books, research updates, conference information Web links, and news. The sections for patients and family members contain articles in lay terms, a frequently asked questions page, downloadable educational coloring books, and locations of sickle cell clinics nationwide. There is an extensive list of links to other sickle cell Web sites. There is a resource page with recommended books, videos, monographs, and CD-ROMs. Worldwide sickle cell educational conferences are posted. There is an informational guide for teachers and employers to help sickle cell patients with basic pain-prevention measures. And there is a free monthly e-mail newsletter subscription on the News page.

Sickle Cell Information Center
P.O. Box 109
Grady Memorial Hospital
80 Jesse Hill Jr. Drive SE
Atlanta, GA 30303
404-616-3572
404-616-5998 fax
www.SCInfo.org

The American Pain Society

This organization has published "The Guideline for the Management of Acute and Chronic Pain in Sickle-Cell Disease" and has many pain-management resources. The "Guideline" is an excellent handbook focusing on pain assessment and treatment. The review is evidence based and peer reviewed by many experts in sickle cell disease.
The American Pain Society
4700 W. Lake Avenue
Glenview, IL 60025
847-375 4715
847-375-6315 fax
www.ampainsoc.org
E-mail: info@ampainsoc.org

Globin Gene Server

This site provides data and tools for studying the function of DNA sequences, with an emphasis on those involved in the production of hemoglobin. There is an online copy of A Syllabus of Human Hemoglobin Variants (1996) and most of A Syllabus of Thalassemia Mutations (1997).
http://globin.cse.psu.edu

Centers for Disease Control (CDC) Sickle Cell Information Web Page
This site has sickle cell information on incidence and prevention of complications.
Centers for Disease Control
1600 Clifton Road
Atlanta, GA 30333
800-232-4636
www.cdc.gov/ncbddd/sicklecell

E-Medicine Health
This site features an electronic medical textbook chapter on sickle cell pain crisis written for healthcare professionals; it has excellent information. www.emedicinehealth.com/sickle_cell_crisis/article_em.htm.
Also see: http://emedicine.medscape.com/article/778971-over-
   view.

Gene Gateway
This site offers a profile of sickle cell disease, from the NIH sickle cell information page.
www.ornl.gov/sci/techresources/Human_Genome/
   posters/chromosome/sca.shtml

Florida Partnership for Access to Sickle Cell Services
This organization, known as PASS, has many resources for sickle cell organizations.
http://floridasickle.org

Genetics Home Reference
This site present information from the NIH on sickle cell disease.
http://ghr.nlm.nih.gov/condition=sicklecelldisease.

University of Rochester Medical Center
This site has brochures and fact sheets on hemoglobinopathies.
www.urmc.rochester.edu/smd/genetics/hemobroc.htm

Sickle Cell Disease Information for School Personnel
An online book for school teachers, nurses, and coaches.
www.state.nj.us/health/fhs/sicklecell

Sickle Cell Kids
This is a kid-friendly site full of sickle cell information in a fun, animated presentation. There are games, stories, letters from celebrities, and more. The staff of the Sickle Cell Center in Atlanta provides the scientific content.
www.SickleCellKids.org

Starlight Children's Foundation
This excellent online resource for children and teens teaches preventive health habits and all about common blood tests, bone marrow, IVs, and x-rays. There is an educational sickle cell quiz game called "Slime-O-Rama" and a social networking site called "Starbright World." This is available for free to patients and families.
www.starlight.org

Harvard School of Medicine Information Center for Sickle Cell and Thalassemic Disorders
This excellent site has information for clinicians and patients. There are very good articles about current issues in sickle cell treatment and links to other sickle cell sites.
http://sickle.bwh.harvard.edu/index.html

March of Dimes
Sickle cell information for professionals can be found at www.marchofdimes.com/professionals/14332_1221.asp.
www.marchofdimes.com

National Library of Medicine

Free Medline searching of the latest publications in the medical press. There are free journal abstracts and many free full-text articles.

www.pubmed.gov

Medline Plus—Sickle Cell Anemia

This site offers many links to sickle cell information.

www.nlm.nih.gov/medlineplus/sicklecellanemia.html

The Virginia Sickle Cell Awareness Program

A complete guide for counseling and education for the most common hemoglobin variants identified through Virginia's sickle cell screening program.

www.vahealth.org/sicklecell/pubssc.htm

Health Hop Medical Rap Music

Sickle Cell Rap Music, Teaching CD—A wonderful teaching tool produced by two family practice physicians, the Clarke brothers, for children and teens. The site offers a CD featuring sickle cell–related rap music and teaches with positive energy. Further information is available from the Clarke brothers.

www.healthhopmusic.com

VIDEOS

You Tube

This online community offers many free educational videos about sickle cell disease and trait. Just type in "sickle cell" in the search box. Any individual can post a video on this site, so it is a powerful way to share your message. Like any thing on the Internet, you must be wary of the sources you watch.

"Living with Sickle Cell Disease," by the Sickle Cell Trust and Dr. Graham Sergeant

A 27-minute VHS video produced in Jamaica. $30. Address: 14 Milverton Crescent, Kingston 6, Jamaica, West Indies. Tel 876-970-0077; Fax 876-970-0074; E-mail: grserjeant@cwjamaica.com.

BOOKS AND BOOKLETS

Understanding Sickle Cell Disease, by Miriam Bloom, Ph.D.

This is an excellent book written for lay audiences by the former senior editor for the Journal of the National Cancer Institute. The book is well organized and contains current information explaining the origins, complications, treatments, and the future of research for sickle cell disease. It is excellent for patients, parents, and lay audiences interested in sickle cell. The book is available from University Press Books, 601-982-1800, and online at www.sciwrite.com/sickle.html.

Sickle Cell Disease, Third Edition, by Graham Serjeant, M.D.

This is one of the most comprehensive medical textbooks in the world. Dr. Serjeant spent much of his medical career caring for sickle cell patients in Jamaica and has traveled around the world as a sickle cell consultant. This text is written for medical personnel, but it is the one reference book to have on the shelf. Oxford Press 2001. ISBN 0-19-263036-9.

Puzzles, by Dava Walker

Puzzles is a story about Cassie, a school-age child with sickle cell disease. This book for children is available from Carolina Wren Press at 919-560-2738. ISBN 0-914996-29-0. There is a 30% discount for schools, hospitals, clinics, libraries, and other nonprofit agencies.

Renaissance of Sickle Cell Disease Research in the Genome Era, edited by Betty S. Pace

This is a wonderful text book for clinical and basic researchers in hematology and genetics, graduate students and postdoctoral fellows; Secondary market: Nursing students, community sickle cell programs, medical school libraries, public library. It has several great authors who are the leaders in sickle cell research and treatment. This book is great for anyone wanting to know the current state of sickle cell disease research. University of Texas at Dallas, ISBN 978-1-86094-645-5 1-86094-645-3. www.worldscibooks.com/lifesci/p443.html.

"Sickle," by Dominique Friend

"Sickle" is a book written by Dominique Friend about her personal experiences living with sickle cell disease. Its purpose is to encourage, uplift, and bring forth awareness of a disease that affects almost 1 in 500 African Americans. Dominique has captured in writing the very essence of what it is like to find purpose in spite of pain, transfusions, medicines, and emergency room visits. Her story will inspire others to speak out and gain confidence "that the battle against this disease does go on." This book is truly a must-have for all those affected by sickle cell disease.

Now You See Me, Now You Don't, by Jan Reed-Givhan

This is a moving and inspiring novel about a young black girl's battle with racial discrimination, as well as sickle cell anemia. Based upon a true story, this book poignantly reveals what challenges a teenage girl can face growing up with a terrible disease, in a sometimes emotionally unhealthy environment. Her story pulls no punches, and yet offers greater understanding and hope.

Ethnicity and Screening for Sickle Cell/Thalassemia, by S. M. Dyson. ISBN 0-443-10232-5. Oxford: Elsevier Churchill Livingston.

Transfusion Support in Patients with Sickle Cell Disease, from the American Association of Blood Banks. The authors of this clinically focused book review the current knowledge and practices in transfusing patients with sickle cell disease to assist clinicians in understanding the complex role transfusion plays in treatment of this disease. 1998; 398 pp., hardbound, ISBN 0-931092-22-1.

Sickle Cell Pain Progress in Pain Research and Management, v. 11, by Samir K. Ballas. 1998; 398 pp., hardbound, ISBN 0-931092-22-1.

"Sickle Cell Disease—A Booklet for Patients, Parents, and the Community," by Dr. Adlette Inati Khoriaty
The objective of this booklet is to provide families of patients affected with sickle cell disease with accurate and concise information about this disease to help them give their children the best treatment possible. This booklet is also meant to enable parents to actively share with their physicians in the care of their children and often suspect the diagnosis of devastating complications and seek help at an early age. It will also help parents handle the disease and teach them ways of dealing with their children in a positive, supportive, and disciplined manner. In addition, this booklet will provide older patients with concise and simplistic information about coping with the disease and its complications. Now available on TIF Web site: www.thalassaemia.org.cy/publications.html.

Uncertain Suffering: Racial Health Care Disparities and Sickle Cell Disease (George Gund Foundation Imprint in African-American Studies), by Carolyn Moxley Rouse
This book provides a richly nuanced examination of what race disparities mean for health care in the United States. Through the lens of sickle cell anemia, Rouse argues that resources should be redirected to community-based health programs that reduce daily forms of physical and mental suffering.

Menace in My Blood: My Affliction with Sickle-Cell Anemia, by Ola Tamedu

Tamedu relates growing up in a fairly well-to-do family in West Africa and highlights the difficulties of life with sickle cell disease. 187 pages; catalogue #04-2825; ISBN 1-4120-5017-0. www.trafford.com/04-2825.

A Guide to Sickle Cell Disease,
by the Sickle Cell Trust and Dr. Graham Serjeant

An 86-page paperback reference with color pictures and guides for common problems. $30. Address: 14 Milverton Crescent, Kingston 6, Jamaica, West Indies. Tel 876-970-0077; Fax 876-970-0074; E-mail: grserjeant@cwjamaica.com.

Overcoming Pain, by Allan Platt, Susan Platt, Cathy Hedrish

An in-depth review of pain management for the layperson. Hilton Publishing, 2005, ISBN 0974314420.

Sickle Cell Disease, by Susan Dudley Gold

A 48-page book for families and older children. The feature of the book is Keon Penn, the first sickle cell patient to undergo unrelated cord blood stem cell transplant. Enslow Publishers, 2001.

Sickle Cell Anemia,
by Alvin and Virginia Silverstein, and Laura Silverstein Nunn

A 112-page book for families and patients. It is easy to read and understand. Enslow Publishers, 1997.

Dying in the City of Blues: Sickle Cell Anemia
and the Politics of Race and Health, by Keith Wailoo

This is a 360-page description of the history, social, cultural, and political aspects of sickle cell disease in Memphis, TN. University of North Carolina Press, 2001.

MEETINGS

There are several national and regional meetings listed on the News page at the Sickle Cell Information Web site at *www.SCInfo. org*. You also can subscribe to the free monthly e-mail newsletters. Some are for patients and families; others are for medical providers. Some offer content for both audiences.

CLINICS

The national and international list of clinics with sickle cell services is growing daily. Please check the latest list on the Sickle Cell Informational website at *www.SCInfo.org/ Clinics.htm*. If you cannot find a clinic near you , ask other patients and supporters about where they obtain good medical care. If you have no patients or sickle cell associations to ask, start with the nearest hematologist, followed by your pediatrician. It is worthwhile to establish annual contact with a large sickle cell center to keep informed about the latest advances and have an established relationship if you have a complicated problem.

SCHOLARSHIPS

A state-by-state listing of member chapters where you can obtain local chapter scholarship information is located at *www.sicklecelldisease.org*.

HEALTH PASSPORT
MEDICAL INFORMATION TO KEEP

Name:_____

Date of Birth:_____

Sickle Cell Type (SS, SC, SBth):_____

Medical Record Number:_____

Allergies:_____

Medications:_____

Physician:_____

Phone:_____

Complications:_____

_____

_____

Transfusions:_____

Surgeries:_____

Pain Medications:_____

ER Pain Medications:_____

APPENDIX I

The History of Sickle Cell Disease

BACKGROUND

Hemoglobinopathies are a group of genetic diseases that occur because of a mutation in the DNA blueprint that directs the making of hemoglobin. Hemoglobin is important because it is the main carrier of oxygen in the body. Only 1 percent of the wide variety of hemoglobinopathies can cause serious diseases such as sickle cell disease and the thalassemias. Thus, you and I can carry a hemoglobin gene abnormality and not know about it because it does not show itself as disease.

Sometimes we take knowledge for granted without honoring the human effort that went into gaining it. Let's correct that by going back in time to see how we learned that hemoglobinopathies are inherited from our parents.

The story begins in the 19th century, when a simple but very damaging blood disorder called *hemophilia* plagued royal families, though only the males were afflicted by it. Hemophilia leads to massive bleeding when an injury occurs inside or outside the body. Without treatment, the hemophiliac can die of bleeding from even minor wounds.

Treatment for hemophilia means transfusion, but blood transfusion wasn't available at this time. And without the benefits of transfusion, most hemophiliacs, even royal ones, easily bled to death.

In 1865, an Austrian monk named Gregor Mendel proposed that discrete units he called *factors* (later to be called *genes)* are passed down among family members to produce particular observable characteristics he called traits.

The scientific community didn't immediately act on Mendel's theory. Part of the problem was the novelty of the ideas. First, Mendel had presented his now famous garden pea experiments in a mathematical model. The math was simple enough, but biologists at that time were not used to interpreting experiments in mathematical terms.

There was a second reason for the gap between Mendel's work and the important work that followed from it. The very concept of cell division, crucial to Mendel's theory, had not yet been discovered. In fact, it was still unknown when Mendel died in 1884. But scientific progress soon changed that, leading to the identification and treatment of genetic diseases, including sickle cell disease.

ONE HUNDRED YEARS OF SICKLE CELL DISEASE RESEARCH AND TREATMENT

Sickle cell disease has probably been in the world for thousands of years. There are African writings that described the symptoms of sickle cell and gave it names like chwecheechwe, abututuo, nuidudui, and nwiiwii. The first published reports of sickle cell disease in African medical literature were in the 1870s.

1910—One hundred years ago, the first well-documented American case of sickle cell disease described was that of Walter Clement Noel, a first-year dental student at the Chicago College of Dental Surgery. Noel, who grew up in Grenada and moved to Chicago to attend dental school, was admitted to the Presbyterian Hospital in late 1904. He had leg ulcers, dizziness, and a breathing problem. Ernest E. Irons, a 27-year-old intern, obtained Noel's history and performed routine physical, blood, and urine examinations. Irons noticed that Noel's blood smear contained "many pear-shaped and elongated forms" and alerted his attending physician, James B. Herrick, to the unusual blood findings. Irons drew a rough sketch of these red blood cells in the hospital record. Herrick and Irons followed Noel over the next two-and-a-half years through several episodes of severe illness. Then Noel returned to Grenada to practice dentistry. He died nine years later at the age of 32 of pneumonia or acute chest syndrome. Herrick published the report "Peculiar elongated and sickle-shaped red blood corpuscles in a case of severe anemia" in the *Archives of Internal Medicine*, volume 6, pages 512–521, in 1910.

In that same year, Thomas Morgan, working at Columbia University, discovered from his research on fruit flies that genes are carried in chromosomes.

1917—V. E. Emmel reported in the *Archives of Internal Medicine* that the sickling observed by James Herrick occurred both in healthy individuals (with sickle trait) and in people who had anemia (sickle cell disease).

1927—Gillespie and Hahn demonstrated that it was a reduction in the oxygen content of the blood that led to the sickling of the red blood cells observed by Herrick. It was Hahn who first used the phrase "sickle cell trait" to describe those healthy individuals who had some sickling of red blood cells but no apparent anemia.

1944—researchers at Rockefeller Institute in New York discovered that genes are made of deoxyribonucleic acid (DNA).

1948—Linus Pauling demonstrated, by comparing normal and sickle hemoglobin, that abnormal hemoglobin was the cause of sickle cell disease. In a paper titled "Sickle Cell Anemia, a Molecular Disease," published in *Science*, he explained how protein electrophoresis was used to show that sickle cell hemoglobin differed in structure from normal hemoglobin. This was the first time that the cause of a disease was linked to a change in protein structure.

1953—James Watson and Francis Crick, working at Cambridge University in England, carried this work a significant step further by uncovering the nature of the DNA molecule itself. The DNA, they noted, contains sugars, phosphates, and bases that are arranged in a spiral, complementary fashion, which they termed the "double helix." The DNA itself, in the nucleus of the molecule, provides a blueprint for the making of protein in the cytoplasm.

1956—Vernon Ingram painstakingly arranged, without benefit of the automated gene sequencers we have today, in their exact order, the amino acids that make up hemoglobin. In this way Ingram showed for the first time that an amino acid called valine had replaced another amino acid called glutamic in the sixth position of the beta globin chain of hemoglobin. This very small change, as we all now know, had very great impact on the lives of people who suffer from it.

1960—Sydney Brenner, Matthew Meselson, and Francois Jacob discovered how information from the DNA in the nucleus is carried into the cytoplasm to make cells, identifying ribonucleic acid (RNA). RNA, coded by the DNA, carries the same configuration as the DNA into the cytoplasm and translates that message in the building of the cells proteins.

1972—Congress passed the National Sickle Cell Anemia Control Act, and the NHLBI established Comprehensive Sickle Cell Centers.

1977—Walter Gilbert and Frederick Sanger developed new techniques for rapid DNA sequencing. This led to the identification of the mutation in the beta globin gene.

1980—The first statewide newborn screening program was implemented to detect sickle cell disease and trait at birth.

1984—The first 24-hour comprehensive sickle cell center opened at Grady Memorial Hospital in Atlanta, Georgia, offering specialized care outside the traditional emergency room.

Also in that year, the first sickle cell patient was cured by bone marrow transplant. By 2009, 276 bone marrow transplants had

had been done, with a 91%–97% survival rate and 7%–10% graft failure rate.

A new treatment option was also introduced in 1984. The medication hydroxyurea was found to increase fetal hemoglobin in sickle cell patients. This discovery has offered promising possibilities. In 1991, Multicenter Study of Hydroxyurea in Sickle Cell Anemia (MSH) began. It was stopped early in 1995 because of proven benefits—reduced pain crisis, reduced hospital admissions, and reduced need for blood transfusions. In 2003, a follow up study reported that patients taking hydroxyurea have a prolonged life. And in 2008, a Consensus Statement from the NIH reported that more patients would benefit from hydroxyurea therapy.

1986—Penicillin Prophylaxis in Sickle Cell Disease, or PROPS, showed that prophylactic administration of penicillin to children from 6 months to age 6 prevents potentially fatal pneumococcal infection.

1987—The NIH held a consensus development conference on Newborn Screening for Sickle Cell Disease and Other Hemoglobinopathies and recommended that "every child should be screened for hemoglobinopathies to prevent the potentially fatal complications of sickle cell disease during infancy." In that year, 14 states were doing newborn screening for sickle cell; by 2002, 44 states did Hb screening, and, by 2009, all 50 states were screening for hemoglobinopathies.

1995—Transfusion guidelines were first published. In surgical settings, simple transfusions to increase hemoglobin (Hb) levels to 10 g/dL are as good as or safer than aggressive transfusions to reduce sickle hemoglobin (Hb S) levels to below 30 percent. Researchers have found that transfusions to maintain a hematocrit of more than 36 percent do not reduce complications of pregnancy.

1997—The Stroke Prevention Trial in Sickle Cell Anemia (STOP) demonstrated that periodic transfusions could prevent first time stroke in susceptible children. Researchers have found that Trans Cranial Doppler Ultrasound (TCD) screening is effective in predicting which children are at highest risk for strokes. All sickle cell disease patients 24 months of age should be screened, and this screening should be repeated every 6–12 months during early childhood.

1997—Investigators inserted the human gene responsible for sickle cell disease into mice, thereby creating transgenic models of the human disease known as Sickle Cell Mice. This breakthrough has led to important new developments. In 2008, scientists at St. Jude's Research Hospital used a harmless virus to insert a corrective gene into mouse blood cells. Via this method, the St. Jude scientists have alleviated sickle cell disease pathology. In their studies, the researchers found that the treated mice showed essentially no difference from normal mice.

1998—Doctors at the AFLAC Cancer Center of Egleston Children's Hospital at Emory University in Atlanta performed the first unrelated donor cord blood stem transplant on Keone Penn, a 12-year-old with sickle cell anemia. He was cured of his sickle cell disease, but he had complications from the transplant.

2000—Pneumococcal conjugate vaccine (PCV), known as Prevnar, was released for immunization. By administering PCV, pneumoccal infections went from1.7 infections per 100 person-years (1995–2000) to 0.5 infections per 100 person-years (2001–2002), which represents a 68% reduction. This has saved lives.

2003—The Human Genome Project was completed. Started in 1990, the U.S. Human Genome Project, coordinated by the U.S. Department of Energy and the National Institutes of Health, identified all the approximately 20,000–25,000 genes in human DNA, and determined the sequences of the 3 billion chemical base pairs.

2005—The FDA approved Exjade (deferasirox), an oral iron chelator, for the treatment of iron overload.

2006—Senators Talent, Schumer, and Burr provided support during African American Health Month by authoring a letter requesting funding in the FY07 Labor/H Appropriations bill to create 40 treatment centers to provide medical treatment and education services for patients living with sickle cell disease. Several senators signed the letter by April 2006, requesting the funding to support the program.

2007—The National Athletic Trainers Association presented its Consensus Statement: Sickle Cell and the Athlete, identifying 13 football player deaths, as well as numerous illnesses and deaths in basketball and distance running. Continuing from these findings, the 2008–09 NCAA Sports Medicine Handbook recommended excluding students with sickle cell disease from serial sprints and performance tests. The handbook recommended that athletes stop if they experience cramps or sudden weakness, or have trouble breathing. The NCAA recommended that athletes train over time but not push past endurance.

June 19, 2009 was the First Sickle Cell Disease World Day at the United Nations, established to bring global awareness and focus on sickle cell disease.

APPENDIX II

Glossary

Acute Chest Syndrome—When sickled red blood cells block blood flow to the lungs. This can cause chest pain, shortness of breath, and cough. It is treated in the hospital with blood transfusions. It can be prevented with incentive spirometry or a blow bottle.

Amniocentesis—A test done by taking a small amount of fluid from the womb of a pregnant woman to determine if the baby has sickle cell disease or another genetic problem. This is usually performed when the pregnancy is 15–18 weeks along.

Anemia—A low red blood cell count. Anemia can be caused by many different events, including sickle cell disease.

Aplastic Anemia or Aplastic Crisis—Decreased red blood cell count due to the bone marrow factory temporarily shutting down. The most common cause is a virus called Parvo B19.

Bone Marrow—The blood factory inside of your big bones that makes red blood cells, white blood cells, and platelets.

Bone Marrow Transplant—A procedure that kills the existing bone marrow factory and plants donor (usually a matched brother or sister) marrow by transfusion. The bone marrow begins to make blood cells according to the genetic code of the donor. This has cured several sickle cell patients.

Carrier—One who inherits only one gene for a genetic problem like sickle cell. Usually there are no symptoms, and the carrier will never have the disease. Two carriers have a 25% risk of having a child with the disease.

Chorionic Villus Sampling (CVS)—This is a procedure to determine if a baby in the womb has a genetic disease like sickle cell. It is done when the pregnancy is 10–12 weeks along. A catheter or needle is used to get a sample of the placenta for testing.

Chromosome—The DNA code for all the parts of the human body. Each person has 46 individual chromosomes in cells, 23 donated from each parent. Chromosome 11 is where the sickle cell mutation occurs.

Complete Blood Count (CBC)—A blood test that gives clinicians information about how many red cells, white cells, and platelets a person has in their bloodstream.

Cord Blood—This is the blood remaining in the umbilical cord and placenta after a baby is born and the cord is cut. This blood is rich in stem cells that can be saved and used in transplants.

Folic Acid or Folate—A B vitamin necessary for making new red blood cells. It also acts as a vasodilator, which allows your blood to flow more freely through small blood vessels, and it helps homocysteine level, which may reduce your risk of complications, such as stroke, leg ulcers, and heart attack. Most sickle cell patients should take 1 mg a day. It is found in green, leafy vegetables, fruits, and whole grains.

Gallbladder—A pouch in the right upper abdomen under the liver. It stores bile to help digest fats in the diet.

Gallstones—Too much bilirubin from red blood cell breakdown can cause stones to form in the gallbladder. This can cause pain in the right upper abdomen, nausea, and indigestion when eating fatty foods. The gallbladder can be removed if it is full of stones.

Genes—These are the basic units of inheritance. They are located on chromosomes.

Gene Therapy—Treatment that will change the genetic defect or the gene product (hemoglobin) in sickle cell disease. This is experimental at this time.

Hand-Foot Syndrome or Dactylitis—Swelling and pain in the hands and feet, usually seen in six-month- to three-year-old sickle cell patients.

Hemoglobin—The protein substance inside the red blood cells that holds and releases oxygen. This is where the sickle mutation occurs.

Hemoglobin Electrophoresis—The blood test that identifies the type of hemoglobins present in the red blood cells.

Hemoglobin AS—This is sickle cell trait. The inheritance of a normal A hemoglobin gene and a sickle hemoglobin gene.

Hemoglobin S Beta Thalassemia—This is a type of sickle cell disease in which one inherits an S gene and a beta thalassemia gene from his or her parents. S beta^0 thalassemia is more severe than S beta$^+$ thalassemia.

Hemoglobin SC—A type of sickle cell disease in which one inherits an S gene and a C gene from the parents. This causes sickle cell complications, with increased eye and bone problems. Life expectancy is longer than with hemoglobin SS.

Hemoglobin SS—This is called sickle cell anemia and is the most common form of sickle cell disease.

Hemolysis—The breaking apart of red blood cells. Normal red cells last 120 days; sickled red blood cells last about fourteen days.

Hydroxyurea—The first medication for sickle cell disease that increases fetal hemoglobin. It reduces pain events by one half, the need for hospital admissions, and the need for blood transfusions—and it prolongs the lifespan.

Intravenous (IV)—A small plastic catheter placed in a vein to allow water, blood, or medication to enter the blood stream directly.

Jaundice—A yellow color in the white part (sclera) of the eye produced by increased bilirubin in the blood. Usually caused by increased red blood cell breakdown in sickle cell patients.

Magnetic Resonance Imaging (MRI)—A large magnet-based device that painlessly creates images of the brain and other organs of the body

Pain Episode or "Crisis"—Pain in the bones and muscles where blood flow has been blocked by sickled red blood cells.

Portacath—An under-the-skin port that requires only a one-time needle stick that allows long-term painless access to sample venous blood, and/or to give IV fluids and medications.

Priapism—A prolonged painful erection of the penis from trapped sickled red blood cells.

Pulmonary Hypertension—The condition in which the lungs' blood vessels are abnormally tight and raise the blood pressure there.

Reticulocyte Count or Retics—The count of brand new red blood cells just released from the bone marrow factory. It is the best indicator of how the bone marrow factory is producing red cells.

Sequestration—Blocked blood flow from sickled red blood cells in the spleen or liver. Blood can flow in, but it cannot flow out. This causes weakness, abdominal pain, and swelling of the liver or spleen.

Spleen—An organ in the left upper area of the stomach that helps filter germs from the blood stream.

Stroke—Blocked blood flow to an area of the brain that can cause weakness, numbness, trouble speaking, or trouble thinking.

Transcranial Doppler (TCD)—a special ultrasound device that uses painless sound waves to check for blocked blood flow in the brain. This test can identify children at greatest risk of having a stroke.

APPENDIX III

Bibliography

Adams, R. J., V. C. McKie, L. Hsu, et al. 1998. Prevention of a first stroke by transfusions in children with sickle cell anemia and abnormal results on transcranial Doppler ultrasonography. *New England Journal of Medicine* 339: 5–11.

Adeodu, O. O., T. Alimi, and A. D. Adekile. 2000. A comprehensive study of the perception of sickle cell anemia by married Nigerian rural and urban women: Complications of sickle cell trait. *West African Journal of Medicine* 19(1): 1–5.

Aldrich, T. K., S. K. Dhuper, W. S. Patwa, E. Makolo, S. M. Suzuka, S. A. Najeebi, S. Santhanakrishnan, R. L. Nagel, and M. E. Fabry. 1996. Pulmonary entrapment of sickle cells: The role of regional alveolar hypoxia. *Journal of Applied Physiology* 80(2): 531–39.

Alegre, M.-L., K. Gastadello, D. Abramovicz, P. Kinnaert, P. Vereerstraeten, L. DePauw, P. Vandenabeele, M. Moser, O. Leo, and M. Goldman. 1991. Evidence that pentoxifylline reduces anti-CD3 monoclonal antibody-induced cytokine release syndrome. *Transplantation* 52(4): 674–79.

Al-Salem, A. H., and S. Oaisruddin. 1998. The significance of biliary sludge in children with sickle cell disease. *Pediatric Surgery International* 13(1): 14–16.

Aluoch, J. R. 1995. The presence of sickle cells in the peripheral blood film: Specificity and sensitivity of diagnosis of homozygous sickle cell disease in Kenya. *Tropical & Geographical Medicine* 47(2): 89–91.

Aluoch, J. R. 1997. Higher resistance to plasmodium falciparum infection in patients with homozygous sickle cell disease in western Kenya. *Tropical Medicine & International Health* 2(6): 568–71.

American College of Physicians. 2008. Summaries for patients: Pain and health care visits in patients with sickle cell disease. *Annals of Internal Medicine* 148(2): I36.

American Medical Association. 1985. Council report: Guidelines for handling parenteral antineoplastics. *Journal of the American Medical Association* 233(11): 1590–92.

American Society of Hospital Pharmacists. 1990. Technical assistance bulletin on handling cytotoxic and hazardous drugs. *American Journal of Hospital Pharmacy* 47: 1033–49.

Angelkort, B. 1979. Thrombozytenfunktion, plasatische blutzerinnung und fibrinolyse bei chronisch aterieller verschluss kranheit. *Die Medizinische Welt* 30: 1239–43.

Angelkort, B., N. Maurin, and K. Booteng. 1979. Influence of pentoxifylline on erythrocyte deformability in peripheral occlusive disease. *Current Medical Research and Opinion* 6: 255–58.

Armitage, J. O. 1998. Bone Marrow Transplantation. In *Harrison's principles of internal medicine*, 14th ed., ed. A. S. Fauci, E. Braunwald, D. L. Kaspar, S. L. Hauser, D. L. Longo, J. L. Jameson, and J. Loscalzo, 724–30. New York: McGraw-Hill.

Assimadi, J. K., A. D. Gbadoe, and M. Nyadanu. 2000. The impact on families of sickle cell disease in Togo. *Archives of Pediatrics & Adolescent Medicine* 7(6): 615–620.

Ataga, K. I., and E. P. Orringer. 2000. Renal abnormalities in sickle cell disease. *American Journal of Hematology* 63(4): 205–11.

Baird, J. K., D. J. Fryauff, H. Basri, M. J. Bangs, B. Subianto, I. Wiady, B. Leksana, S. Masbar, T. L. Richie, T. R. Jones, E. Tjitra, S. Wignall, and S. L. Hoffman. 1995. Primaquine for prophylaxis among nonimmune transmigrants in Irian Java, Indonesia. *American Journal of Tropical Medicine and Hygiene* 52(6): 479–84.

Ballas, S. K. 2009. The cost of health care for patients with sickle cell disease. *American Journal of Hematology* 84(6): p. 320–22.

Ballas, S. K., and N. Mohandas. 1996. Pathophysiology of vaso-occlusion. *Hematology/Oncology Clinics of North America* 10: 1221–39.

Behrens, R. J., and T. C. Cymet. 2000. Sickle cell disorders: Evaluation, treatment, and natural history. *Hospital Physician* 36: 9.

Belgrave, F. Z., and S. D. Molock. 1991. The role of depression in hospital admissions and emergency treatment of patients with sickle cell disease. *Journal of the National Medical Association* 83(9): 777–81.

Bellet, P. S., K. A. Kalinyak, R. Shukla, M. J. Gelfand, D. L. Rucknagel. 1995. Incentive spirometry to prevent acute pulmonary complications in sickle cell diseases. *New England Journal of Medicine* 333(11): 699–703.

Benjamin, G. C. 1993. Sickle cell anemia. In *The Cambridge world history of human disease*, ed. K. F. Kiple, 1006–07. Cambridge, U.K.: Cambridge University Press.

Benjamin, L. J., et al. 1999. Guideline for the management of acute and chronic pain in sickle cell disease—American Pain Society clinical practice guidelines series, no. 1. Glenview, Ill.: American Pain Society.

Beutler, E. 1995. The sickle cell diseases and related disorders. In *Williams hematology*, 5th ed., ed. E. Beutler, et al., 616–54. New York: McGraw-Hill.

Beutler, E. 1998. Disorders of hemoglobin. In *Harrison's principles of internal medicine*, 14th ed., ed. A. S. Fauci, E. Braunwald, D. L. Kaspar, S. L. Hauser, D. L. Longo, J. L. Jameson, and J. Loscalzo, 645–52. New York: McGraw-Hill.

Bitanga, E., and J. D. Rouillon. 1998. Influence of sickle cell trait on energy and abilities. *Pathologie Biologie (Paris)* 46(1): 46–52.

Bloom, M. 1999. *Understanding sickle cell disease.* Jackson, Miss.: University Press of Mississippi.

Boogaerts, M. A., S. Milbrain, P. Meerus, L. van Hove, and G. E. G. Verhoef. 1990. In vitro modulation of normal human neutrophil function by pentoxifylline. *Blut* 61: 60–65.

Brawley, O. W., et al. 2008. National Institutes of Health consensus development conference statement: Hydroxyurea treatment for sickle cell disease. *Annals of Internal Medicine* 148(12): 932–38.

Bruno, D., D. R. Wigfall, S. A. Zimmerman, P. M. Rosoff, and J. S. Wiener. 2001. Genitourinary complications of sickle cell disease. *Journal of Urology* 166(3): 803–11.

Bunn, H. F. 1997. Pathogenesis and treatment of sickle cell disease. *New England Journal of Medicine* 337: 762–69.

Burlew, K., J. Telfair, L. Colangelo, and E. L. Wright. 2000. Factors that influence adolescent adaptation to sickle cell disease. *Journal of Pediatric Psychology* 25(5): 287–99.

Cao, A. 1994. 1993 William Allan Award address. *American Journal of Human Genetics* 54: 397–402.

Cartwright, K. 1995. Meningococcal carriage and disease. In *Meningococcal disease*, ed. K. Cartwright, 115–46. Chichester, U.K.: John Wiley & Sons.

Castro, O., D. J. Brambilla, B. Thorington, et al. 1994. The acute chest syndrome in sickle cell disease: Incidence and risk factors—The cooperative study of sickle cell disease. *Blood* 84(2):643–49.

Centers for Disease Control and Prevention. 1996. Health information for international travelers: HHS pub. no. 96–8280. Washington, D.C.: U.S. Department of Health and Human Services.

Centers for Disease Control and Prevention. 1998. Mortality among children with sickle cell disease identified by newborn screening during 1990–1994—California, Illinois, and New York. *Morbidity and Mortality Weekly Report* 47(9): 169–72.

Cepeda, M. L., F. H. Allen, N. J. Cepeda, and Y. M. Yang. 2000. Physical growth, sexual maturation, body image, and sickle cell disease. *Journal of the National Medical Association* 92(1): 10–14.

Chambers, J. B., D. A. Forsythe, S. L. Betrano, H. J. Iwinski, and D. E. Steflik. 2000. Retrospective review of osteoarticular in a pediatric sickle cell age group. *Journal of Pediatric Orthopaedics* 20(5): 682–85.

Chang, Y. P., M. Maier-Redelsperger, K. D. Smith, et al. 1997. The relative importance of the X-linked FCP locus and beta-globin haplotypes in determining haemoglobin F levels: A study of SS patients homozygous for beta S haplotypes. *British Journal of Haematology* 96(4): 806–14.

Chao, N. J., S. M. Schmidt, J. C. Niland, M. D. Amylon, A. C. Dagis, G. N. Long, A. P. Nadananee, R. S. Negron, M. R. O'Donnell, P. M. Parker, E. P. Smith, D. S. Snyder, A. S. Stein, R. M. Wong, K. G. Blume, and S. J. Forman. 1993. Cyclosporine, methotrexate, and prednisone compared with cyclosporine and prednisone for prophylaxis of acute graft-vs-host disease. *New England Journal of Medicine* 329: 1225–30.

Charache, S., F. B. Barton, R. D. Moore, M. L. Terrin, M. H. Steinberg, G. J. Dover, S. K. Ballas, R. P. McMahon, O. Castro, and E. P. Orringer. 1996. Hydroxyurea and sickle cell anemia: Clinical utility of a myelosuppressive 'switching' agent—The multicenter study of hydroxyurea in sickle cell anemia. *Medicine* 75(6):300–326.

Charache, S., G. J. Dover, R. D. Moore, S. Eckert, S. K. Ballas, M. Koshy, P. F. Millner, E. P. Orringer, G. Phillips Jr., O. S. Platt, and G. U. Thomas. 1992. Hydroxyurea: Effects on hemoglobin F production in patients with sickle cell anemia. *Blood* 79: 2555–65.

Charache, S., M. L. Terrin, R. D. Moore, et al. 1995. Effect of hydroxyurea on the frequency of painful crises in sickle cell anemia. *New England Journal of Medicine* 332: 1317–22.

Chinegwundoh, F., and K. A. Anie. 2004. Treatments for priapism in boys and men with sickle cell disease. *Cochrane Database of Systematic Reviews* 18(4): CD004198.

Cipolotti, R., M. F. Caskey, et al. 2000. Childhood and adolescent growth of patients with sickle cell disease in Aracaju, Sergipe, north-east Brazil. *Annals of Tropical Paediatrics* 20(2): 109–13.

Clark, C. 1998. Gene therapy: A promising strategy for sickle cell anemia. *Blood Weekly* (June 22), 13.

Clift, R. A., C. D. Bucker, F. R. Appelbaum, G. Schoch, F. B. Peterson, W. I. Bensinger, W. J. Senders, R. M. Sullivan, R. Storb, and J. Singer. 1992. Allogeneic marrow transplantation during untreated first relapse of acute myeloid leukemia. *Journal of Clinical Oncology* 10: 1723–29.

Clinical Oncological Society of Australia. 1983. Guidelines and recommendations for safe handling of antineoplastic agents. *Medical Journal of Australia* 1: 426–28.

Consensus Conference. 1987. Newborn screening for sickle cell disease and other hemoglobinopathies. *Journal of the American Medical Association* 258(9): 1205–09.

Crystal, R. G. 1995. Transfer of genes to humans: Early lessons and obstacles to success. *Science* 270: 404–10.

Davies, S. M., X. O. Shu, B. R. Blazar, A. H. Filipovich, J. H. Kersey, W. Krivit, J. McCullough, W. J. Miller, N. K. C. Ramsay, M. Segall, J. E. Wagner, D. J. Weisdorf, and P. B. McGlave. 1995. Unrelated donor bone marrow transplantation: Influence of HLA A and B incompatibility on outcome. *Blood* 86: 1636–42.

Davis, H., R. M. Moore Jr., and P. J. Gergen. 1997. Cost of hospitalizations associated with sickle cell disease in the United States. *Public Health Reports* 112(1): 40–43.

Derchi, G., G. L. Forni, F. Formisano, M. D. Cappellini, R. Galanello, G. D'Ascola, P. Bina, C. Magnano, and M. Lamagna. 2005. Efficacy and safety of sildenafil in the treatment of severe pulmonary hypertension in patients with hemoglobinopathies. *Haematologica* 90(4): 452–58.

Dormandy, J., G. B. Nash, T. Loosemore, and P. R. Thomas. 1990. Effects of acute trental on white cell rheology in patients with critical leg ischemia. In *Pentoxifylline and analogues: Effects on leukocyte function*, ed. J. Hakim, G. L. Mandell, and W. J. Novick Jr., 203–05. Basel, Switzerland: S. Karger.

Eckman, J. R. 2001. Techniques for blood administration in sickle cell patients. *Seminars in Hematology* 38(1, Suppl 1): 23–29.

Eckman, J. R., and A. F. Platt. 1991, 2002. Problem oriented management of sickle cell syndromes, 4th ed: NIH pub. no. 02-2117. Bethesda, Md.: National Institutes of Health, National Heart, Lung, and Blood Center. Available online at www.scinfo.org/ index.php?option=com_content&view=category&id=15:the-management-of-sickle-cell-disease-4th-ed&Itemid=5.

Egrie, J. C., T. W. Strickland, J. Lane, K. Aoki, A. M. Cohen, R. Smalling, G. Trail, F. K. Lin, J. K. Browne, and D. K. Hines. 1986. Characterization and biological effects of recombinant human erythropoietin. *Immunobiology* 172: 213–24.

Ehlers, K. H., P. J. Giardina, M. L. Lesser, M. A. Engle, and M. W. Hilgartner. 1991. Prolonged survival in patients with beta-thalassemia treated with deferoxamine. *Journal of Pediatrics* 118: 540–45.

Embury, S. H., J. F. Garcia, N. Mohandas, R. Pennathur-Das, and M. R. Clark. 1984. Effects of oxygen inhalation on endogenous erythropoietin kinetics, erythropoiesis, and properties of blood cells in sickle-cell anemia. *New England Journal of Medicine* 311: 291–95.

Embury, S. H., R. P. Hebbel, and N. Mohandas, eds. 1994. *Sickle cell diseases: Basic principles and clinical practice*. Hagerstown, Md.: Lippincott-Raven.

Eschbach, J. W., J. C. Egrie, M. R. Downing, J. K. Browne, and J. W. Adamson. 1987. Correction of the anemia of end-stage renal disease with recombinant human erythropoietin. *New England Journal of Medicine* 316(2): 73–78.

Eschbach, J. W., J. C. Egrie, M. R. Downing, J. K. Browne, and J. W. Adamson. 1989. The use of recombinant human erythropoietin (r-HuEPO): Effect in end-stage renal disease (ESRD). In *Prevention of chronic uremia*, ed. E. A. Friedman, M. Boyer, N. G. DeSanto, and C. Giordano, 148–55. Philadelphia: Field and Wood Inc.

Fedson, D. S., and D. M. Musher. 1994. Pneumococcal vaccine. In *Vaccines*, 2d ed., ed. S. A. Plotkin and E. A. Mortimer Jr., 517. Philadelphia: Saunders.

Ferrari, E., M. Fioravanti, A. L. Patti, and C. Viola. 1987. Effects of long-term treatment (four years) with pentoxifylline on hemor-rheological changes and vascular complications in diabetic patients. *Pharmatherapeutica* 5: 26–39.

Field, J. J., J. E. Knight-Perry, and M. R. Debaun. 2009. Acute pain in children and adults with sickle cell disease: Management in the absence of evidence-based guidelines. *Current Opinion in Hematology* 16(3): 173 78.

Firth, P. G., and R. A. Peterfreund. 2000. Management of multiple intra-cranial aneurysms: Neuroanesthetic considerations of sickle cell disease. *Journal of Neurosurgical Anesthesiology* 12(4): 366–71.

Fitzgerald, R. K., and A. Johnson. 2001. Pulse oximetry in sickle cell ane-mia. *Critical Care Medicine* 29(9): 1803–06.

Fitzhugh, C. D., D. R. Wigfall, and R. E. Ware. 2005. Enalapril and hydroxyurea therapy for children with sickle nephropathy. *Pediatric Blood & Cancer* 45: 982–85.

Fleming, D. R., N. K. Rayens, and J. Garrison. 1997. Impact of obesity on allogeneic stem cell transplant patients: A matched case-controlled study. *American Journal of Medicine* 102(3): 265–68.

Frasch, C. E. 1995. Meningococcal vaccines: Past, present, and future. In *Meningococcal disease*, ed. K. Cartwright, 35–70. Chichester, U.K.: John Wiley & Sons.

Gaston, M. H, J. L. Verter, G. Woods, et al. 1986. Prophylaxis with oral penicillin in children with sickle cell anemia: A randomized trial. *New England Journal of Medicine* 314: 1593–99.

Gill, F. M., L. A. Sleeper, S. J. Weiner, et al. 1995. Clinical events in the first decade in a cohort of infants with sickle cell disease—The coopera-tive study of sickle cell disease. *Blood* 86(2): 776–83.

Glickman, E., M. M. Horowitz, R. E. Chanopin, J. M. Hows, A. Bacigalapo, J. L. Biggs, B. M. Camitta, R. P. Gale, L. C. Gordon-Smith, A. M. Marmont, T. Masuoka, N. K. C. Ramsay, A. Rima, C. Rozman, K. A. Sabocinski, B. Speck, and M. M. Bortin. 1992. Bone marrow transplantation for severe aplastic anemia: Influence of conditioning and severe graft-vs-host disease prophylaxis regimens on outcome. *Blood* 79: 269–75.

Godeau, B., F. Galacteros, A. Schaeffer, F. Morinet, D. Bachir, J. Rosa, and J. L. Portos. 1991. Aplastic crisis due to extensive bone marrow necrosis and human parvovirus infection in sickle cell disease. *American Journal of Medicine* 91(5): 557–58.

Goldstein, M. 1999. *The Nature of Animal Healing*. New York: Alfred A Knopf.

Graber, S. E., and S. B. Krantz. 1978. Erythropoietin and the control of red cell production. *Annual Review of Medicine* 29: 51–58.

Grant, M. M., K. M. Gill, M. Y. Floyd, and M. Abrams. 2000. Depression and functioning in relation to health care use in sickle cell disease. *Annals of Behavioral Medicine* 22(2): 149–57.

Gucalp, R., and J. Dutcher. 1998. Oncologic Emergencies. In *Harrison's principles of internal medicine*, 14th ed., ed. A. S. Fauci, E. Braunwald, D. L. Kaspar, S. L. Hauser, D. L. Longo, J. L. Jameson, and J. Loscalzo, 627–34. New York: McGraw-Hill.

Hassell, K. L., J. R. Eckman, and P. A. Lane. 1994. Acute multiorgan failure syndrome: A potentially catastrophic complication of severe sickle cell pain episodes. *American Journal of Medicine* 96(2): 155–62.

Hassell, K. L., B. Pace, W. Wang, R. Kulkarni, C. S. Johnson, J. Eckman, P. A. Lane, W. G. Woods, and American Society of Pediatric Hematology/Oncology. 2009. Sickle cell disease summit: From clinical and research disparity to action. *American Journal of Hematology* 84(1): 39–45.

Hillman, R. S. 1998. Iron deficiency and other hypoproliferative anemias. In *Harrison's principles of internal medicine*, 14th ed., ed. A. S. Fauci, E. Braunwald, D. L. Kaspar, S. L. Hauser, D. L. Longo, J. L. Jameson, and J. Loscalzo, 638–45. New York: McGraw-Hill.

Hiruma, H., C. T. Noguchi, N. Uyesaka, S. Hasegawa, E. J. Blanchette-Mackie, A. N. Schecter, and G. P. Rodgers. 1995. Sickle cell rheology is determined by polymer fraction—Not cell morphology. *American Journal of Hematology* 48(1): 19–28.

Human Genome Program. 2008. Gene therapy. In *Human genome project information*. Oak Ridge, Tenn.: U.S. Department of Energy, Office of Biological and Environmental Research. Available at: www.ornl.gov/sci/techresources/Human_Genome/medicine/genetherapy.shtml.

Ibidapo, M. O., and O. O. Akinyaju. 2000. Acute sickle cell syndromes in Nigerian adults. *Clinical and Laboratory Haematology* 22(3): 151–55.

Israel, R. A., H. M. Rosenberg, and L. R. Curtin.1986. Analytical potential for multiple cause-of death data. *American Journal of Epidemiology* 124: 161–79.

Itoh, T., S. Chien, and S. Usami. 1995. Effects of hemoglobin concentration on individual sickle cells after deoxygenation. *Blood* 85: 2245–53.

Jean-Baptiste, G. A., and K. Leuleer. 2000. Osteoarticular disorders of hematological origin. *Baillière's Best Practice & Research Clinical Rheumatology* 14(2): 307–23.

Jim, R. T. S. 1988. New therapy for microangiopathic hemolytic anemia caused by cardiac valve prosthesis: A case report. *Hawaii Medical Journal* 47: 285.

Johnson, C., ed. 2005. Sickle cell disease: Special issue. *Hematology/Oncology Clinics of North America* 19(5): 771–996.

Jones, R. B., R. Frank, and T. Mass. 1983. Safe handling of chemotherapeutic agents: A report from the Mount Sinai Medical Center. *CA: A Cancer Journal for Clinicians* 33(5): 258–63.

Kachmaryk, M. M., S. N. Trimble, and R. G. Gieser. 1995. Cilioretinal artery occlusion in sickle cell trait. *Retina* 15: 501–04.

Kark, J. A., D. M. Posey, H. R. Schumacher, and C. J. Ruehle. 1987. Sickle-cell trait as a risk factor for sudden death in physical training. *New England Journal of Medicine* 317: 781–86.

Kerle, K. K., and K. D. Nishimura. 1996. Exertional collapse and sudden death associated with sickle cell trait. *American Family Physician* 54(1): 237–40.

King, A. A., D. A. White, R. C. McKinstry, M. Noetzel, and M. R. DeBaun. 2007. A pilot randomized education rehabilitation trial is feasible in sickle cell and strokes. *Neurology* 68(23): 2008–11.

Kinney, T. R., R. W. Helms, E. E. O'Branski, K. Ohen-Frempong, W. Wang, C. Daeschner, E. Vichinsky, R. Redding-Lallinger, B. Gee, O. S. Platt, and R. E. Ware. 1999. Safety of hydroxyurea in children with sickle cell anemia: Results of the HUG-KIDS study, a phase I/II trial—Pediatric Hydroxyurea Group. *Blood* 94(5): 1550–54.

Krause, P. J., K. G. Maderazo, J. Contrino, L. Eisenfeld, V. C. Herson, N. Greca, P. Bannon, and D. L. Kreutzer. 1991. Modulation of neonatal neutrophil function by pentoxifylline. *Pediatric Research* 29: 123–27.

Krishnamurti, L. 2007. Hematopoietic cell transplantation: A curative option for sickle cell disease. *Journal of Pediatric Hematology/Oncology* 24(8): 569–75.

Ladwig, P., and H. Murray. 2000. Sickle cell disease in pregnancy. *Australian and New Zealand Journal of Obstetrics and Gynaecology* 40(1): 97–100.

Lanzkron, S., C. Haywood Jr., J. B. Segal, and G. J. Dover. 2006. Hospitalization rates and costs of care of patients with sickle-cell anemia in the state of Maryland in the era of hydroxyurea. *American Journal of Hematology* 81(12): 927–32.

Leiken, S. L., D. Gallagher, T. R. Kinney, et al. 1989. Mortality in children and adolescents with sickle cell disease—The cooperative study of sickle cell disease. *Pediatrics* 84(3): 500–508.

Lell, B., J. May, and R. J. Schmidt. 1999. The role of red blood cell polymorphism in resistance and susceptibility to malaria. *Clinical Infectious Diseases* 28(4): 794–99.

Leonhardt, H., and H.-G. Grigoleit. 1977. Effects of pentoxifylline on red blood cell deformability and blood viscosity under hyperosmolar conditions. *Naunyn-Schniedeberg's Archives of Pharmacology* 299: 197–200.

Lorey, F. W., J. Arnopp, and G. Cunningham. 1996. Distribution of hemoglobinopathy variants by ethnicity in a multiethnic state. *Genetic Epidemiology* 13: 501–512.

Lorey, F. W., G. Cunningham, F. Shafer, B. Lubin, and E. Vichinsky. 1994. Universal screening for hemoglobinopathies using high-performance liquid chromatography: Clinical results of 2.2 million screens. *European Journal of Human Genetics* 2: 262–71.

Lucarelli, G., M. Galimberti, P. Polchi, E. Angelucci, D. Barancianci, C. Giardini, P. Politi, S. M. Durazzi, P. Muretto, and F. Albertini. 1990. Bone marrow transplantation in patients with thalassemia. *New England Journal of Medicine* 322: 417–21.

Lundin, A. P., M. J. H. Akerman, and R. M. Chester. 1991. Exercise in hemodialysis patients after treatment with recombinant human erythropoietin. *Nephron* 58: 315–19.

Machado, R. F., S. Martyr, G. J. Kato, R. J. Barst, A. Anthi, M. R. Robinson, L. Hunter, W. Coles, J. Nichols, C. Hunter, V. Sachdev, O. Castro, and M. T. Gladwin. 2005. Sildenafil therapy in patients with sickle cell disease and pulmonary hypertension. *British Journal of Haematology* 130(3): 445–53.

Manci, E. A., D. E. Culberson, Y. M. Yang, T. M. Gardner, R. Powell, J. Haynes Jr., A. K. Shah, and V. N. Mankad. 2003. Investigators of the cooperative study of sickle cell disease—Causes of death in sickle cell disease: An autopsy study. *British Journal of Haematology* 123(2): 359–65.

Marshall, E. 1995. Gene therapy's growing pains. *Science* 269: 1050–55.

Medical Economics. 1999. *Physicians' desk reference*, 53d ed. Montvale, N.J.: Medical Economics Inc.

Meshikhes, A.-W. N., S. A. al-Dhurais, A. al-Jama, et al. 1995. Laparoscopic cholecystectomy in patients with sickle cell disease. *Journal of the Royal College of Surgeons of Edinburgh* 40: 383–85.

Michlitsch, J. G., and M. C. Walters. 2008. Recent advances in bone marrow transplantation in hemoglobinopathies. *Current Molecular Medicine* 8(7). 675–89.

Mohan, J. S., J. E. Vigilance, J. M. Marshall, I. R. Hambleton, H. L. Reid, and G. R. Serjeany. 2000. Abnormal venous function in patients with homozygous sickle cell (SS) disease and chronic leg ulcers. *Clinical Science (Colchester)* 98(6): 667–72.

Morris, C. R., G. J. Kato, M. Poljakovic, X. Wang, W. C. Blackwelder, V. Sachdev, S. L. Hazen, E. P. Vichinsky, S. M. Morris Jr., and M. T. Gladwin. 2005. Dysregulated arginine metabolism, hemolysis-associated pulmonary hypertension, and mortality in sickle cell disease. *Journal of the American Medical Association* 294(1): 81–90.

Morris, C. R. 2009. Asthma management: Reinventing the wheel in sickle cell disease. *American Journal of Hematology* 84(4): 234–41.

Müller, R. 1981. Hemorheology and peripheral vascular disease: A new therapeutic approach. *Journal of Medicine* 12(4): 209–35.

Musher, D. M. 1998. Pneumococcal Infections. In *Harrison's principles of internal medicine*, 14th ed., ed. A. S. Fauci, E. Braunwald, D. L. Kaspar, S. L. Hauser, D. L. Longo, J. L. Jameson, and J. Loscalzo, 869–75. New York: McGraw-Hill.

Nagel, R. L., and H. M. Ranney. 1990. Genetic epidemiology of structural mutations of the beta-globin gene. *Seminars in Hematology* 27(4): 342–59.

National Center for Biotechnology Information. 1998. Hemoglobin—Beta locus; HBB: Online Mendelian inheritance in man (OMIM). MIM no. 141900. Baltimore, Md.: The Johns Hopkins University. Available at: www.ncbi.nlm.nih.gov/omim/141900.

National Heart, Lung, and Blood Institute. 2010. Collection and storage of umbilical cord stem cells for treatment of sickle cell disease. Bethesda, Md.: National Institutes of Health. Available online at: http://clinicaltrials.gov/NCT00012545.

National Human Genome Research Institute. 2010. Learning about sickle cell disease. Bethesda, Md.: National Institutes of Health. Available at: www.genome.gov/10001219.

National Institutes of Mental Health. 1983. Recommendations for the safe handling of parenteral antineoplastic drugs: NIH pub. no. 83–2621. Washington, D.C.: U.S. Department of Health and Human Services.

National Study Commission on Cytotoxic Exposure. 1987. Recommendations for handling cytotoxic agents. Boston: Massachusetts College of Pharmacy and Allied Health Sciences.

Neonato, M. G., M. Guillod-Batalle, P. Beauvais, P. Beguei P, et al. 2000. Acute clinical events in 299 homozygous sickle cell patients living in France—French study group on sickle cell disease. *European Journal of Haematology* 65(3): 155–64.

New York Newsday. 1999. Briefs. *New York Newsday*, 1 Dec.: A38.

Newborn Screening Committee, The Council of Regional Networks for Genetic Services (CORN). 1998. National newborn screening report—1993. Atlanta: CORN.

Nietert, P. J., M. R. Abboud, M. D. Silverstein, and S. M. Jackson. 2000. Bone marrow transplantation versus periodic prophylactic blood transfusion in sickle cell patients at high risk of ischemic stroke: A decision analysis. *Blood* 95(10): 3057–64.

Nissenson, A. R., S. D. Nimer, and D. L. Wolcott. 1991. Recombinant human erythropoietin and renal anemia: Molecular biology, clinical efficacy, and nervous system effects. *Annals of Internal Medicine* 114(5): 402–16.

Norris, W. E. 2004. Acute hepatic sequestration in sickle cell disease. *Journal of the American Medical Association* 96(9): 1235–39.

Nwadiaro, H. C., B. T. Ugwu, and J. N. Legbo. 2000. Chronic osteomyelitis in patients with sickle cell disease. *East African Medical Journal* 77(1): 23–26.

Occupational Safety and Health Administration. 1996. Controlling occupational exposure to hazardous drugs: OSHA work practice guidelines. *American Journal of Health-System Pharmacy* 53: 1669–85.

Office of Science Policy. 2009. About Recombinant DNA Advisory Committee (RAC). In *Office of Biotechnology activities*. Bethesda, Md.: National Institutes of Health. Available at: http://oba.od.nih.gov/rdna_rac/rac_about.html.

Ogandi, S. O., and F. Onwe. 2000. A pilot survey comparing the level of sickle cell disease knowledge in a university of south Texas and a university in Enugu, Enugu state, Nigeria, West Africa. *Ethnicity and Disease* 10(2): 232–36.

Ohene-Frempong, K. 2001. Indications for red cell transfusion in sickle cell disease. *Seminars in Hematology* 38(1 Suppl 1): 5–13.

Ohene-Frempong, K., S. J. Weiner, L. A. Sleeper, et al. 1998. Cerebrovascular accidents in sickle cell disease: Rates and risk factors. *Blood* 91(1): 288–94.

Oyesiku, N. M., J. R. Eckman, D. L. Barrow, S. C. Tindall, and A. R. Colohan. 1991. Intracranial aneurysms in sickle cell anemia: Clinical features and pathogenesis. *Journal of Neurosurgery* 75(3): 356–63.

Paciocco, G., F. J. Martinez, E. Bossone, E. Pielsticker, B. Gillespie, and M. Rubenfire. 2001. Oxygen desaturation on the six-minute walk test and mortality in untreated primary pulmonary hypertension. *European Respiratory Journal* 17(4): 647–52.

Pack-Mabien, A., and J. Haynes Jr. 2009. A primary care provider's guide to preventive and acute care management of adults and children with sickle cell disease. *Journal of the American Academy of Nurse Practitioners* 21(5): 250–57.

Platt, O. S., D. J. Brambilla, W. F. Rosse, et al. 1994. Mortality in sickle cell disease: Life expectancy and risk factors for early death. *New England Journal of Medicine* 330(23): 1639–44.

Platt, O. S., B. D. Thorington, D. J. Brambilla, et al. 1991. Pain in sickle-cell disease—Rates and risk factors. *New England Journal of Medicine* 325: 11–16.

Porter, J. B. 2007. Concepts and goals in the management of transfusional iron overload. *American Journal of Hematology* 82(12 Suppl): 1136–39.

Powars, D., and A. Hiti. 1993. Sickle cell anemia: Beta s gene cluster haplotypes as genetic markers for severe disease expression. *American Journal of Diseases of Children* 147(11): 1197–1202.

Prabhakar, H. 2009. Improving the quality of care for sickle cell disease for patients and providers in the United States: A review of general considerations and observations for improving health systems management of sickle cell disease. Baltimore, Md.: The Johns Hopkins University.

Rahimy, M. C., A. Gangboa, R. Adjou, C. Deguenon, S. Goussanou, and E. Ahihonou. 2000. Effect of active management on pregnancy outcome in sickle cell disease in an African setting. *Blood* 96(5): 1685–89.

Reed, W., and E. P. Vichinsky. 2001. Transfusion therapy: A coming-of-age treatment for patients with sickle cell disease. *Journal of Pediatric Hematology/Oncology* 23(4): 197–202.

Sacerdote, A. 1999. Treatment of homozygous sickle cell disease with pent-oxifylline. *Journal of the National Medical Association* 91(9): 466–70.

Sacerdote, A., and A. Bishnoi. 1989. Enhanced reduction of proteinuria in diabetics with triple therapy: Pentoxifylline, protein restriction, and angiotensin converting enzyme inhibitors. *Diabetes* 38(supp): 158A.

Sacerdote, A., and A. Bishnoi. 1989. Triple therapy for proteinuria in diabetics; Pentoxifylline, protein restriction, and angiotensin converting enzyme inhibitors. *Clinical Research* 37: 860A.

Sacerdote, A., and M. Rodriguez. 1994. Treatment of homozygous SS disease with pentoxifylline. *Clinical Research* 42: 239A.

Schnetterer, L., D. Kemmler, H. Breitenender, C. Alschinger, R. Koppensteiner, F. Lexer, A. F. Fercher, H. Eichler, and M. Wolgt. 1996. A randomized, placebo-controlled, double-blind crossover of the effect of pentoxifylline on ocular fundus pulsations. *American Journal of Opthalmology* 121: 169–76.

Schubert, T. T. 1986. Hepatobiliary system in sickle cell disease. *Gastroenterology* 90: 2013.

Schubolz, R., and O. Mufellner. 1977. The effect of pentoxifylline on erythrocyte deformability and phosphatide fatty acid distribution in the erythrocyte membrane. *Current Medical Research and Opinion* 4: 609–17.

Segal, M. 1989. New hope for children with sickle cell disease. *FDA Consumer* (March): 14–19.

Serjeant, G. R. 1997. Sickle cell disease. *Lancet* 350: 725–30.

Shanks, G. D. 1995. Malaria prevention and prophylaxis. In *Ballière's clinical infectious diseases*, vol. 2, ed. G. Pasvol, 331–49. London, U.K.: Ballière Tindall.

Shapiro, E. D., A. T. Berg, R. Austrian, D. Schroeder, V. Parcells, A. Margolis, R. K. Adair, and J. D. Clemens. 1991. The protective efficacy of polyvalent pneumococcal polysaccharide vaccine. *New England Journal of Medicine* 325: 1453–60.

Sickle Cell Disease Guideline Panel. 1993. Sickle cell disease: Screening, diagnosis, management, and counseling in newborns and infants—Clinical practice guideline no. 6 (AHCPR pub. no. 93–0562). Rockville, Md.: Agency for Health Care Policy and Research, Public Health Service, U.S. Department of Health and Human Services.

Silverstein, A., V. B. Silverstein, and L. S. Nunn. 1997. *Sickle cell anemia.* Springfield, N.J.: Enslow Publishers, Inc.

Simberkoff, M. S., A. P. Cross, M. Al-Ibrahim, A. L. Baltch, P. J. Geiseler, J. Nadler, A. S. Richmond, R. P. Smith, G. Schiffman, D. S. Shepard, J. P. Van Eeckhout. 1986. Efficacy of pneumococcal vaccine in high-risk patients: Results of a Veteran Administration cooperative study. *New England Journal of Medicine* 315(21): 1318–27.

Snyder, H. W., A. Mittelman, A. Oral, G. L. Messerschmidt, D. H. Henry, S. Korec, J. H. Bertran, T. H. Guthrie Jr., D. Ciarella, D. Wuest, W. Perkins, J. P. Balint Jr., S. K. Cochran, R. Pengout, and F. R. Jones. 1993. Treatment of cancer chemotherapy-associated thrombotic thrombocytopenic/hemolytic uremic syndrome by protein A immunoadsorption of plasma. *Cancer* 71(5):1882–92.

Solanki, D. L., G. G. Kletter, O. Castro. 1986. Acute splenic sequestration crises in adults with sickle cell disease. *American Journal of Medicine* 80(5): 985–90.

Solberg, C. O. 1998. Meningococcal infections. In *Principles of internal medicine*, 14th ed., ed. A. S. Fauci, E. Braunwald, D. L. Kaspar, S. L. Hauser, D. L. Longo, J. L. Jameson, and J. Loscalzo, 910–15. New York: McGraw-Hill.

Solerte, S. B., and E. Ferrari. 1985. Diabetic retinal vascular complications and erythrocyte flexibility: Results of a two-year follow-up study with pentoxifylline. *Pharmatherapeutica* 4: 341–49.

Steinberg, M. H. 1999. Management of sickle cell disease. *New England Journal of Medicine* 340: 1021–30.

Steinberg, M. H., F. Barton, O. Castro, et al. 2003. Effect of hydroxyurea on mortality and morbidity in adult sickle cell anemia: Risks and benefits up to 9 years of treatment. *Journal of the American Medical Association* 289(13): 1645–51.

Steketee, R. W., J. J. Wirima, L. Slutsker, C. O. Khoromana, D. L. Heymann, and J. G. Breman. 1996. Malaria treatment and prevention in pregnancy: The indications for use and adverse events associated with use of chloroquine and mefloquine. *American Journal of Tropical Medicine and Hygiene* 55(1 suppl): 50–56.

Stuart, M., R. Nagel. 2004. Sickle cell disease. *Lancet* 364: 1323–60.

Styles, L. A., and E. Vichinsky. 1994. Effects of a long-term transfusion regimen on sickle cell-related illnesses. *Journal of Pediatrics* 125: 909–11.

Thomas, P. W., D. R. Higgs, and G. R. Serjeant. 1997. Benign clinical course in homozygous sickle cell disease: A search for predictors. *Journal of Clinical Epidemiology* 50(2): 121–26.

Treacy, E., B. Childs, and C. R. Scriver. 1995. Response to treatment in hereditary metabolic disease. *American Journal of Human Genetics* 56(2):359–67.

University of Texas Health Science Center. 1995. Pathophysiology and management of sickle cell pain crisis: Report of a meeting of physicians and scientists, University of Texas Health Science Center at Houston, Texas. *Lancet* 346: 1408–11.

U.S. Public Law 92-294. National sickle cell anemia control act of 1972. *U.S. Statutes at Large* 86: 138.

Valle, D. 1998. Treatment and prevention of genetic disease. In *Harrison's principles of internal medicine*, 14th ed., ed. A. S. Fauci, E. Braunwald, D. L. Kaspar, S. L. Hauser, D. L. Longo, J. L. Jameson, and J. Loscalzo, 403–09. New York: McGraw-Hill.

Vichinsky, E. P. 2002. New therapies in sickle cell disease. *Lancet* 360(9333): 629–31.

Vichinsky, E. P., C. M. Haberkern, L. D. Neumayr, et al. 1995. A comparison of conservative and aggressive transfusion regimens in the perioperative management of sickle cell disease. *New England Journal of Medicine* 333: 206–13.

Vichinsky, E. P., L. D. Neumayr, A. N. Earles, R. Williams, E. T. Lennette, D. Dean, B. Nickerson, E. Orringer, V. McKie, R. Bellevue, C. Daeschner, and E. A. Manci. 2000. Causes and outcomes of the acute chest syndrome in sickle cell disease—National acute chest syndrome study group. *New England Journal of Medicine* 342(25): 1855–65.

Vichinsky, E. P., O. Onyekwere, J. Porter, P. Swerdlow, et al. 2007. A randomised comparison of deferasirox versus deferoxamine for the treatment of transfusional iron overload in sickle cell disease. *British Journal of Haematology* 136(3): 501–08.

Wahl, S., and K. C. Quirolo. 2009. Current issues in blood transfusion for sickle cell disease. *Current Opinion in Pediatrics* 21(1): 15–21.

Walters, M. C., K. Ohene-Frempong, M. Patience, W. Leisenring, J. R. Eckman, J. P. Scott, W. C. Mentzer, S. C. Davies, F. Bernandin, D. C. Matthews, R. Storb, and K. M. Sullivan. 1996. Bone marrow transplantation for sickle cell disease. *New England Journal of Medicine* 335: 369–76.

Walters, M. C., M. Patience, W. Leisenring, et al. 1997. Collaborative multicenter investigation of marrow transplantation for sickle cell disease: Current results and future directions. *Biology of Blood and Marrow Transplantation* 3: 310–15.

Wang, W. C., R. W. Helms, H. S. Lynn, R. Redding-Lallinger, B. E. Gee, K. Ohene-Frempong, K. Smith-Whitley, M. A. Waclawiw, E. P. Vichinsky, L. A. Styles, R. E. Ware, and T. R. Kinney. 2002. Effect of hydroxyurea on growth in children with sickle cell anemia: Results of the HUG-KIDS study. *Journal of Pediatrics* 140(2): 225–29.

Wethers, D. L. 2000. Sickle cell disease in childhood, part II: Diagnosis and treatment of major complications; Recent advances in treatment. *American Family Physicians* 62(6): 1309–14.

Wikipedia. 2010. Introduction to genetics. In *Wikipedia: The free encyclopedia*. St. Petersburg, Fla.: Wikipedia. Available at: http://en.wikipedia.org/wiki/Introduction_to_Genetics.

Wison Schaeffer, J. J., K. M. Gil, M. Burchinal, K. D. Kramer, K. B. Nash, E. Orringer, and D. Strayhorn. 1999. Depression, disease severity, and sickle cell disease. *Journal of Behavioral Medicine* 22(2): 115–26.

Wun, T., T. Paglieroni, C. L. Field, J. Welborn, A. Cheung, N. J. Walker, and F. Tablin. 1999. Platelet-erythrocyte adhesion in sickle cell disease. *Journal of Investigative Medicine* 47(3): 121–27.

Xu, K., Z. M. Shi, L. L. Veeck, M. R. Hughes, and Z. Rosenwaks. 1999. First unaffected pregnancy using preimplantation genetic diagnosis for sickle cell anemia. *Journal of the American Medical Association* 281: 1701–06.

Yardley-Jones, A. 1999. What are the implications of sickle cell anemia? *Occupational Medicine (London)* 49(1): 55–56.

Yoon, S. L., and A. Godwin. 2007. Enhancing self-management in children with sickle cell disease through playing a CD-ROM educational game: A pilot study. *Pediatric Nursing* 33(1): 60–63, 72.

Zimmerman, S. A., and R. E. Ware. 2000. Palpable splenomegaly in children with hemoglobin SC disease: Hematological and clinical manifestations. *Clinical and Laboratory Haematology* 22(3): 145–56.

INDEX